PLAY GOLF
FOREVER

A physiotherapist's guide to golf
fitness and health for the over 50s

SUZANNE CLARK

Play Golf Forever

First published in 2016 by

Panoma Press Ltd
48 St Vincent Drive, St Albans, Herts, AL1 5SJ, UK
info@panomapress.com
www.panomapress.com

Book design and layout by Neil Coe.

Printed on acid-free paper from managed forests.

ISBN 978-1-784520-87-8

DISCLAIMER

The information in this book is provided for informational purposes only and is not a substitute for professional medical advice. The reader is advised to consult an appropriate healthcare professional regarding all aspects of individual health care. The author and publisher make no legal claims, expressed or implied, and the material in this book is not to replace the services of a healthcare professional. The author, publisher and/or copyright holder assumes no responsibility for the loss or damage caused, or allegedly caused, directly or indirectly by the use of information contained in this book. Individuals who suffer from any disease or are recovering from an injury of any sort should consult their doctor regarding the advisability of undertaking any of the exercises and/or treatment regimes suggested in this book. The author and publisher specifically disclaim any liability incurred from the use or application of the contents of this book.

All contents of this book were accurate and up to date at the time of printing.

TESTIMONIALS

"PGF has helped improve my balance and fitness for everyday things as well as golf. I'm recommending it to all of my golfing friends."

C ROGERS

"The advice on injury prevention and treatment is like having your own personal physio looking after you."

R DAVIS

"This book has given me back my confidence on the golf course with better balance and stronger muscles. I feel like I did years ago!"

M DEVEREUX

ACKNOWLEDGEMENTS

I would like to thank all of my family and friends who have encouraged and supported me whilst writing this book.

In particular, my excellent test readers Howard, Clare and my lovely husband Stacey.

Thank you to my ever patient models, Barry and Natalie and to my photographer Ed.

To Maureen, you are an inspiration to all 'older' golfers and all those who meet you. Thank you for your help and friendship.

The biggest thank you to Nicki. Without your expertise, guidance and understanding, this book would not have been written. You are a fantastic physio and a very dear friend.

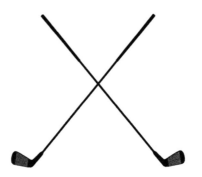

CONTENTS

INTRODUCTION

Play Golf Forever is part of the "Play Forever" series aimed at helping the over 50s stay fitter and healthier in order to enjoy their sport or leisure activity. Following on from *Play Tennis Forever*, a group of avid golfers in their 60s asked me to write a version to help them continue to play and enjoy golf for as long as possible.

This was great in theory, except for one small problem... I'm not a golfer. I wondered if I could begin to understand this very addictive, enjoyable, frustrating game that so many over 50s play.

After studying the biomechanics of golf, walking golf courses with groups of players of all ages and talking to many, many golfers (you can find out a lot about golfing aches and pains at the 19th hole!), I felt that, as a physiotherapist, I could offer valuable advice to this group of sportsmen and women.

Play Golf Forever will help you understand how to make the most of your body. By using easy, targeted exercise, and making simple adaptations in technique or equipment to overcome aches and pains, it will enable you to perform to the best of your ability.

As was the case when researching *Play Tennis Forever*, talking to 'older' golfers highlighted the fact that most people don't understand the ageing process of their bodies. As you get older, your muscles can lose around 1% muscle mass a year from the age of 30 unless you specifically exercise them. With the right kind of exercise you can easily slow this process. It is never too late to start, and the more you do the 'younger' your muscles become. This will keep you playing the sport you love, improve your game through better body conditioning and help avoid injury. You will also gain many secondary health benefits... a win-win... and hopefully more winning on the golf course too!

Talking to people who had given up playing golf, I found that many had stopped playing due to aches and pains that they put down to their age as if it were inevitable. Having met some 90 year old golfers, I don't believe in the 'just getting too old to play'. With some exercise, sometimes a change in equipment and maybe a change in technique, it is possible to adapt to accommodate many limiting factors and, for the younger player, prevent them before they become game limiting. Well worth a try if it keeps you on the golf course.

Most clubs I visited had some 80 year olds and a few had a couple of 90 year olds still playing, and playing well. The thing they all had in common was they had very good technique. This meant less strain on their bodies over the years which enabled them to continue playing. For them age is not an issue, and it doesn't have to be for you.

Golf can be broken down into three categories from a physiotherapist's point of view:

muscle power, flexibility and balance

The simple exercises I recommend will show how you can work on all three easily in your home and that no expensive equipment is needed.

I will not offer any coaching on technique... I'll leave that to your club professionals. However, the better your strength, range of movement (flexibility) and balance, the more you will get out of any coaching sessions you take part in.

All explanations are in simple layman's terms and include a description of what happens to your muscles as you age. I think it is important to understand a little about how your muscles work, especially as you get older, as it gives you an appreciation of why these exercises are key to keeping fitter and younger. Understanding ageing muscle has driven the latest research into best practice for exercise, and the reasons why it is never too late to benefit from a suitable exercise programme. As a physiotherapist I know how boring exercise can be unless you're the type who already hangs out in the gym 3-5 times a week. Consequently, I have devised a programme that you can undertake during everyday activities at home such as watching TV, brushing your teeth, going up stairs. With a little adaptation of these tasks, you can work on your strength, flexibility and balance.

Golf is a very one-sided game for your body, taking your joints repeatedly through the same path of movement. This can cause muscle imbalance and uneven loading on your joints, both of which can cause premature degenerative changes, such as arthritis. In fact, professional golfers were the first sports players to realise this and take their own physiotherapist on tour with them to help avoid these dangers and maintain their fitness and health.

As nice as it would be to have your own personal physiotherapist come round the course with you, and I would love that job, it's just not going to happen for most of us. So, with this book, you will be able to look after yourself to make the most of what you've got, avoid some of the negative effects of golf on your body, slow or prevent your muscles ageing and avoid some common injuries that would otherwise keep you from playing.

There are some common injuries which are experienced by golfers in particular. I will explain what these are and how you can avoid them. I will help you decide if you need to make any small changes to your golfing equipment, maybe have a session with your pro to tweak your technique enough to change stress points in your body, or seek medical advice.

The main message that I want to get across is injury prevention. This is by far the most important aspect for any sports player. Understanding what is necessary to keep your body fit and healthy enough to stand up to the rigors of your sport is the key to a long and productive sporting life. I have therefore included a chapter on injury prevention techniques that will hopefully become second nature to you, keeping you on the golf course, and keeping you healthier for all the activities you undertake.

Remember, your body will not keep itself fit on its own. Golf is a wonderful sport, as you walk a few miles each time you play, but unless you specifically address the wasting in your muscles and the muscle imbalance from the repeated golf swing, your fitness levels will decline as you get older.

My advice is:

Using the suggested exercises, set yourself up with a programme that suits you, in your home, that you can do at least three times a week. The aim is for it to become part of your daily activities so it doesn't seem like hard work and will therefore get done! It really is a case of, 'if you don't use it, you will lose it'.

You will learn how to do your own simple warm-up at home or at your club before you play to help avoid injury and how to cool down after play to keep your muscles flexible.

Understanding the common injuries will help you avoid them. If you do get injured, you will understand the best way to treat yourself and when you need to see a healthcare professional for advice. Ignoring an injury will lead to greater problems in the future with re-injury. The right sort of treatment/rehabilitation will help you get back to golf sooner and safer.

A little work now will be an investment for your playing longevity, and who wants to say later on in life, 'If only I had kept myself a bit fitter?'. A 50, 60 or 70 year old knee will always be a 50, 60 or 70 year old knee, but you can do so much to make it the best 50 to 70 year old knee it can be.

Be fitter, younger and healthier, and you will then get the most out of your golf for many years to come.

CHAPTER 1

HOW YOUR MUSCLES AGE

We all know that our bodies get older, and sometimes they feel older, but what actually happens to your muscles and can you do anything to stop the changes?

The answer is, 'Yes you can'. Inevitably there will be a degree of muscle loss as you get older, in some part due to your lifestyle changing as you age. Often people become more sedentary, probably sitting more than they used to, which will contribute to a loss in muscle mass. It may be medication related depending on what treatments you may be having, or it may directly result from disease. However, there is no reason why you can't minimise or help prevent the loss of muscle mass due to ageing and inactivity with simple exercises. Although there is an abundance of scientific research to support this, many people don't realise:

1. That there is a gradual loss of muscle fibres, medically called *sarcopenia*, from the age of 30 onwards. It is so gradual that you really don't start to notice it until after you are 50, maybe even into your 60s, when you begin to experience the loss in the form of less speed, strength, balance and even loss of muscle bulk.

2. You can minimise the effects of *sarcopenia* with simple exercises that you can do at home. They need to be resistive exercises, meaning that you need to work on the power/strength of the muscles rather than their endurance.

3. You need to do these exercises regularly, initially to build your strength and then as a maintenance programme to keep your muscles strong. If you stop exercising, the muscles will revert to losing strength and muscle fibres.

Sarcopenia: This is the medical term meaning loss of skeletal muscle mass and strength with age. It comes from the Greek meaning 'vanishing flesh' or 'poverty of flesh'. There is an actual decrease in the number of certain muscle fibres and a decrease in the synthesis of the proteins that make muscle. The nerve units, called motor units, decline and so the brain cannot tell the muscle to contract with as much power. A decrease in some hormone levels is also thought to enhance the muscle loss.

I have always been a keen sports player and becoming a physiotherapist was my ticket to understanding how to keep my body as young and fit as I could so that I could carry on playing sport for all of my life. Obviously, qualifying at the age of 21, at that time getting old probably meant 30 plus in my mind. Well, I've now passed 50 and I'm still fit, actively playing sports and taking part in sprint triathlons, and it hasn't been hard to achieve with regular exercise.

There is a myth that once you pass a certain age you can't make your muscles stronger or can't improve your coordination and balance. A friend said to me that I had better start writing my book soon as she was fast approaching 70 and it would then be too late to build any muscles or improve her strength. I realised that this misconception is fairly common which means that many of our mature sports colleagues are slowly declining in their sporting abilities unnecessarily. It is such a shame as there are things that you can do to help prevent it.

People of any age can increase strength and endurance, both of which will not only improve their sporting ability but also have many additional health benefits.

So what part of our muscles do we begin to lose but can get back with simple exercises?

Firstly I need to explain a bit about how our muscles are structured. Our muscles are basically made up of two types of muscle fibres:

Type I which are called 'slow fibres' and Type II which are called 'fast fibres'.

Slow muscle fibres are responsible for endurance; they don't tire so easily but are less powerful. For example, our postural muscles are mainly slow muscle fibres. They need to be strong enough to hold us up against gravity but we don't want them to get tired too quickly or we will have to keep lying down. They are mainly designed for endurance.

Fast fibres are the ones that give us strength. They are powerful but tire quickly. They also make the muscle 'bulky'.

Picture the long distance runner. He requires lots of endurance and most likely has a skinny physique. The 100 metre sprinter requires lots of power for quick bursts of speed and so will be very muscular. The main difference between the training of the two runners is that the long distance runner will do a lot of *aerobic* training, i.e. running rather than spending time lifting weights, so that his heart and lungs work extremely efficiently to get the oxygen to the muscles. He is mainly working on his slow muscle fibres. The sprinter will spend a lot of time in the gym lifting weights, building the power in his muscles, working on his fast muscle fibres. This is called *anaerobic* exercise.

Aerobic exercise: *this is exercise that increases the need for oxygen for the muscles to work. As you breathe you supply the oxygen to the muscles giving them the energy they need to perform. It is also called cardio exercise. It is exercise that is low intensity but can go on for a long time. Walking, slow gentle running and cycling all exercise the slow muscle fibres. Basically, it is any exercise that doesn't require short intensive bursts of power.*

Anaerobic exercise: *this type of exercise does not require oxygen as the muscles get their energy from glycogen which you store ready for use. It is more powerful, and we use this type of exercise when we want bursts of power and strength as in the sprinter or the weight lifter who work their fast muscle fibres. The length of time you can perform anaerobic exercise is much shorter than aerobic exercise as the body uses up the fuel quickly and builds up waste products like lactic acid.*

I'm not advocating that we should all put on our lycra shorts and head to the nearest gym! It is really easy to do some simple anaerobic exercises at home that will help to maintain those fast muscle fibres. If you work them enough, you will be able to increase their number, get stronger and prevent your muscles wasting.

What happens to your muscle fibres as you get older?

You now know about how your muscles are made up and how the different types of exercise work on the different fibres, but what happens to these fibres as we get older?

Studies have shown that from the age of 30 our muscles start to change. We begin to lose muscle mass. We don't notice the muscle loss as it is gradual and does not impair function initially. However, by the time you are 60 you may start to notice it beginning to affect you, and by the time you reach 70 you could have lost between 30% and 40% of your muscle mass or strength if you have not addressed this with appropriate exercise.

That's quite difficult for a keen sportsman to read who wants to carry on playing as if he were still 30. However, a mountain of research backs up the theory that if you regularly perform even modest strengthening exercises you can strongly influence the muscle loss.

One example is shown by a study carried out at a university in Boston, USA (Ref: Physical Therapy January 2002 vol 82 no1 62-68).

The scientists worked with a group of 85-97 year olds. They measured the strength of their quadriceps muscles (the muscles on the front of your thigh) and found that after three months of resisted exercise training (anaerobic exercise) for three sessions a week, their quadriceps strength had improved on average by 134%. Amazing! So, no excuses, at any age you can start exercising. It is never too late to get fit, build your strength and be healthier for it.

Anaerobic/resisted exercises can:

- Increase the number of fast muscle fibres and thus increase strength.

- Increase the rate that the body synthesises the muscle *proteins* and *hormones*.

- Stimulate the neurological processes to be more efficient/faster, since nerves going to the muscles adapt as demands are made of them.

- Speed up reaction time.

- Also have a positive effect on osteoporosis, as loading a bone through a greater force from a muscle helps to keep it strong.

Proteins: Muscles are made up of two types of protein, actin and myosin, which are basically amino acids that are linked together. So if you are trying to maintain or build more muscle, you will need to provide your body with the amino acids. When we eat proteins such as fish and eggs our bodies break them down into the amino acids which can then help build more actin and myosin.

Hormones: *These are basically chemicals that your brain tells specialist glands to secrete in order to tell different systems in your body what to do. Insulin, testosterone and cortisol all play an important role in exercise and muscle building.*

So you can see that anaerobic (resisted) exercising is essential in maintaining the strength and power of your muscles which will enable you to continue to hit the ball with power and, as your muscles will be quicker to react, have better balance and coordination. Anaerobic exercise helps to reverse the effects of sarcopenia as we age.

Aerobic Exercise

We must remember that aerobic exercising plays a part too, as all forms of exercise have a role to play in our fitness. Aerobic exercises are activities such as walking, cycling and long slow runs. Aerobic exercise works to enlarge the slow muscle fibres which become thinner or smaller as we age. A brisk walk daily is a good aerobic workout.

If you do no aerobic exercise, you will start to lose the endurance of your muscles, such as your postural muscles. Think of an older, non-sporting person you know who has started to become round shouldered and who says they can't walk as far as they used to as they get tired sooner. This is partially a result of their postural muscles losing some of their endurance, causing them to tire sooner. It is a gradual process and they probably didn't notice it creeping up on them. Their posture is generally due to deterioration of their slow muscle fibres, and they tire quickly as the blood supply to the muscles is diminished and the *enzymes* used to convert oxygen to fuel have decreased.

Enzymes: *These are specialist proteins that your body uses to speed up chemical reactions when changing one substance into another.*

Aerobic exercising can:

- Increase the size of the slow muscle fibres

- Increase the blood flow

- Increase the number of fuel cells that provide energy to the muscles (*mitochondria*)

- Increase the oxygen conversion to provide energy

- Decrease fatigue

Mitochondria: *These specialist cells convert the energy in our food into the type of energy that our cells can use to power our muscles. They are really the batteries of our bodies. Studies show that aerobic exercise can increase the number of mitochondria.*

That sounds a bit scientific and daunting, but all you have to do to maintain your aerobic activity is to carry on playing golf as you will be walking a few miles each round. It is said that 45 minutes a day is sufficient, and you will be achieving that already on days when you play. However, there's no harm in doing a little more. Take the stairs rather than the lift. If you can take a brisk walk rather than taking the car, then do so. All these things add up to help minimise the changes. If for some reason you can't play golf for a while, then, if possible, walk. Don't sit and wait, because if you don't use it, you will lose it!

People have said to me, 'But I do yoga every week, isn't that enough?' or, 'But I walk a lot playing golf, doesn't that keep me fit?' They are both great forms of exercise to help in your overall fitness. Yoga helps to maintain flexibility and aid core stability, very important in injury prevention and swing technique, and walking is a good aerobic activity. However, these aren't anaerobic exercises (the strengthening exercises for those fast muscle fibres). This is because yoga does not offer enough resistance to strengthen your muscles. Unless you do specific resisted exercises that work your fast muscle fibres you will lose them. If you walked up and down hills all the time, this type of walking would be giving more resistance to your muscles, but not many of us live on top of a hill!

An important message of this book is that you only have one body, so you need to look after it, and it is not enough just to play your sport if you want to maximise your muscle function. If you want to keep playing for longer, and perform better, then it is best to do some regular resisted exercises. You can also improve the quality of your golf swing with targeted strength training, and don't forget that you will also get huge additional health benefits, such as:

- Increased muscle strength will help protect your joints from arthritic changes.

- Taking your joints through their full range of movement will provide the whole joint surface with nutrition which will also help prevent arthritic changes.

- Preventing shortening of your muscles. Shortened muscles affect their function and predispose your joints to arthritic changes and your muscles to injury.

- Improving reaction time for coordination which in turn improves balance.

- Improved reactions means fewer falls, especially later in life, so there is less chance of fractures.

- A stronger pull of your muscle on bone which can help minimise osteoporotic changes (when your bones become weaker and fragile).

- You will feel more energetic, tire less quickly and so be able to be more active.

- Increased metabolism which helps burn fatty deposits.

One last point that relates to keeping your muscles strong and is important for you as a sports player to understand is: as you get older you begin to lose the water content of your tendons. They basically become more brittle and this puts them at greater risk of injury. The stronger and more flexible your muscles are, the less stress will be put through your tendons. It is so important to prevent injury because it can take longer for older tendons to heal, and the more brittle they are, the less able they are to heal back to 100% performance.

With this in mind, I have worked out a resistance training programme that is appropriate for the older golf player and can be fitted in to your everyday life. You do not have to set aside regular times for exercise if you don't want to – very few people are that dedicated to exercising regularly without getting bored.

The programme also has minimal cost. Sometimes you will be using your body weight as resistance, your stairs and a chair as equipment, or a resistive exercise band and/or small weights. The band and weights will provide resistance through the range of movement of the exercise. This will help strengthen all of the muscles in the same patterns of movement that you use when playing golf.

Biomechanically, meaning how efficiently your body moves, you should be able to swing your club with more power, less fatigue and fewer injuries. Hopefully, you will have a longer playing career as you will stay stronger and fitter.

CHAPTER 2

HOW YOUR MUSCLES WORK WHEN YOU PLAY GOLF

What muscles do we need for golf?

The answer is, you need all of them, but there are a few muscles that you particularly need to keep strong, flexible and balanced to allow you to play the best golf you can. I won't name them all but I will tell you about the main ones you use and why you should keep them strong for your golfing technique.

The exercises I suggest will work these groups of muscles whilst you are doing your daily activities (more on that in Chapter 5, 'Home Exercise Programme'). These muscles are also the ones that are prone to injury as you put the most stress through them during play, so it is really important to keep them strong to help avoid injuries.

The main muscle groups are:

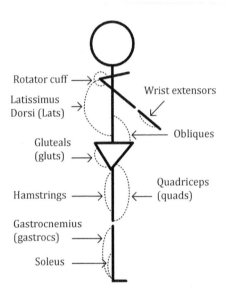

Why are these muscles important for golf? Well, starting from the feet up you need:

- A good base to balance on and push up from… here, the ones you need are the calf muscles (gastrocnemius and soleus) as they help to transfer your weight forward onto your toes which lifts your heels up. You can see this during the golf swing but you also need these muscles for walking the course, especially if the ground is uneven. The muscles are attached to your foot by the Achilles tendon and you will have heard of people 'pulling' their calf muscles or having 'Achilles tendon problems'.

- Strength to control your knees... this is provided by the thigh muscles (quadriceps) on the front and the hamstrings on the back. It is important to keep your quadriceps strong as they are the power house of your movement and they provide around 80% of the stability to your knees. If they get weak, this puts more stress on your knee, predisposing it to arthritic changes. During a technically good golf swing, you use your quadriceps to help generate some of the power to the swing through something called the 'kinetic link' or 'chain' (which I will explain later). On the back of your thighs are the hamstrings which bend your knee and work with the quadriceps to produce stability to your knee in a smooth and controlled way. Many sports players have experienced hamstring injuries and this is partly because the hamstrings are weaker than the quadriceps and so tire more quickly which can make them prone to injury.

- Strength around your hips for stability... and also to keep your pelvis at the right level. There are many muscles around the hips that work together and are responsible for more than one movement, but the gluteal muscles ('gluts') are one of the most powerful muscle groups of the hip. Keeping these strong will help provide stability and power throughout your swing and good alignment of your pelvis and hips which, again, will help minimise stress through your knees. Professional golf players have some of the strongest hip muscles of all sports players.

Moving up to your body:

- 'Core stability' is a trendy term, but what is it? Well, this refers to having strength in all your tummy muscles and back to give you stability and help balance through your body when you move. In golf, you use your core to balance, and you also use the muscles in your tummy that go diagonally across it which are called 'the obliques'. These muscles help to rotate the body and are crucial for the rotational aspect of the swing. One group of back muscles that is also very important for your swing is your latissimus dorsi muscles ('lats'). These run from your shoulder right the way down each side of your spine to the mid-level of your back. These important golf muscles, together with your obliques, are groups of muscles that most recreational players would not necessarily know about and therefore may not include in an exercise regime.

- The shoulders are complicated but obviously very important for the golf player. The shoulder is a fairly unstable joint. We rely on the shoulder ligaments and muscles (rotator cuff is the collective term) to keep the joint functioning correctly. Keeping the muscles strong around the shoulder is one of the best ways to protect it from injury, and increasing their strength will add to your control when hitting the ball. Also, your pectoral muscles ('pecs') connect the shoulder joint to your sternum (chest bone). They play a big part in aiding the swing of your club during rotation of the body, making it a smooth, effective swing.

- Your arms are obviously vital. The forearm muscles that control the wrist are key to holding the club correctly throughout the swing. You will be aware of the term 'golfer's elbow' which is basically inflammation of the tendons joining some of these muscles to the elbow. Keeping these muscles strong will help prevent the stresses on the tendon and help prevent golfer's elbow

That is a very simplified introduction to the main muscle groups that you should be keeping strong in order to play well and prevent injuries. You will find the exercises which will achieve this in Chapter 5, 'Home Exercise Programme'.

How do you coordinate all of the muscles for golf?

Coordinating our muscles is a very important part of learning to play, improving play and for effective rehabilitation following injury. However, it can be overlooked. A basic knowledge of how our muscles are coordinated will enable you to understand how to produce a fluid and efficient movement, why coaching helps improve technique and the importance of specific post-injury exercises.

Muscles do not work in isolation and so need to be coordinated for useful/functional movement to occur. How does this happen? Basically the brain is in charge. It is an amazing organ that coordinates each group of muscles, exactly as we need, to produce a smooth and efficient movement... or so we would like to think when playing golf! You can see how a newcomer to the sport struggles at first to produce a smooth and coordinated swing and their movements are not effortless. This is because the brain is learning what movement patterns are needed and how much effort each muscle has to put in, or not, in order for it to become a smooth movement. When you watch the professionals, don't they make it look easy? That is because they only use the amount of effort required, no more, no less. Their brains have learnt how much contraction, relaxation and coordination between muscle groups is required to create a smooth, fluid and effective movement. We do that with walking. When you watch a toddler learning to walk, their brain is in the process of learning what muscles to use, how much to contract or relax them and which ones they need. It takes a toddler a while before their walking pattern becomes smooth and effortless. Adults don't even think about walking as it is a learned pattern and is automatic. It is efficient and only uses the exact amount of energy needed to perform the task, no more, no less.

When we learn a new skill as an adult, we can analyse and actively adjust what we are doing, so this helps us learn more quickly. Once we begin to experience what the correct swing feels like, we start to learn it, and eventually, with enough practice, reproduce it automatically.

It is never too late for your brain to learn new movement patterns so age is not an excuse to stop learning. Relating this to golf, although you may have got into some bad habits with your swing, it is never too late to learn how to do it properly. It may take a bit longer as old habits die hard, but it is possible and will save you energy, make you a more efficient player and possibly prevent some injuries that are caused by poor technique. Better technique certainly puts less stress through your joints thus keeping them healthier.

Relating this to rehabilitation after an injury, you need to teach the brain and any injury-affected muscles to work in coordination with your other muscles again. That is why physiotherapists always include exercises that work your balance, coordination, and *proprioception* (also called joint position sense) after injury.

> **Proprioception**: *this is the 'body position sense'. If you close your eyes you know what position your body is in, whether your knees are bent or your arms straight. You don't have to look at them to know. This is called proprioception.*

MUSCLE POWER

The importance of muscle strength for golf

You now know what the important muscle groups are. Obviously the more fast fibres these muscles have, the greater the muscle strength. The greater the strength, the more control and power your swing will have.

Once the correct pattern of movement to produce the swing is learnt, it is the '*kinetic link*' that puts it all together and transmits the power created in your muscles up through your body, ending in your hands as they make impact with the ball through the club.

Kinetic link or chain

Kinetic link is a bit of sporty/physiotherapy jargon, and basically refers to the whole movement pattern of the swing from bottom to top (feet to hands), making full use of the power of all of the muscles in the pattern. The power that is generated in the muscles is passed up through to the point of impact, i.e. hitting the ball with not just the power of the muscles in your arm, but also the power of the muscles in your legs and torso.

The kinetic link through the body

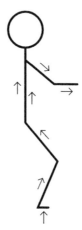

> ***Kinetic link/chain***: *the power generated in the muscles of your feet is transmitted up through your calves, adding their strength, up through your quads, adding their strength, through your trunk, shoulders, arms, and then all of the power is transmitted at the point of impact = when you hit the ball. Thus, no one muscle is responsible for generating the power... it's a team effort!*

The golf swing isn't just a question of standing still and hitting the ball using only your arm and shoulder muscles. A good swing will involve every muscle in your body acting in a coordinated way to give you the balance, stability, power and control where you need it. Power from your gastrocs, quadriceps, gluteal, abdominals (including your obliques) and back muscles, as well as your arm and shoulder muscles, produce the power. That's how good players are able to hit the ball so hard and far. It is a whole chain of sequential movements from your feet up to your head, passing the power through each segment in the most efficient way. If one element goes, the link is broken and the swing will not be efficient or as effective, or it will rely purely on your arm strength. This puts stress through your muscles and tendons in your effort to hit the ball just as hard. You have probably experienced days when you are not hitting the ball so well. You start trying to hit the ball harder using the strength in your arms, rather than the smooth, almost effortless movement of good technique, when the movement flows easily through your body. It is a different feeling altogether.

The difference between when a shot feels right and when it doesn't is when it did not flow through the kinetic link correctly. It is never too late to learn a better movement pattern, and the better shape your muscles are in then the easier it is to learn. If you have some existing medical condition that makes it difficult for you to produce an efficient kinetic chain of movement, then you will probably have learnt to adapt to the most efficient one that you can produce.

Your club professional can analyse your swing and help you to produce your best swing. Admittedly, you will have to keep practising the pattern of movement before it becomes automatic, but practise can be fun and rewarding when it starts going right. To give you a time frame, it can take about 6-8 weeks for your nervous system and your muscles to adapt fully once you start an exercise programme. Be patient and the fruits of your labours will start to show.

I've talked a little about patterns of movement and coordinating your muscles to generate power, but what are the other key skills that are important to enable you to play better golf?

BALANCE

The importance of balance when playing golf

People generally don't think about their balance until they lose it. You just accept that when you get older your balance deteriorates, but with a bit of exercise you can help prevent a lot of this deterioration whatever your age. A friend who recently turned 50 told me that she noticed that she now tended to hold onto something when putting her socks on. This shows that her balance has become less effective and she hadn't realised it despite being a regular tennis player. She started to do simple balance exercises, and after three weeks she was standing unaided to put her socks on... it really can be as simple as that!

Age does affect balance as we rely on our muscles being strong and quick enough to react when our brains tell them to contract in order to maintain balance. If our muscles aren't up to it, then no matter what the brain tells them, they won't react in time and you will lose your balance. Improving your balance, therefore, is another compelling reason to exercise and get those fast muscle fibres working with strength and speed. Resisted exercises together with a simple balance exercise will do this.

The better your balance, the more stable, coordinated and efficient your swing will be. This not only produces a better drive, but also puts less strain through your body. Good balance is fundamental to all sports, and don't forget it will help you in everyday life too, especially as you get older.

FLEXIBILITY

The importance of flexible muscles for golf

The opposite of good flexibility is tight, shortened muscles. In order to understand how to make the most of your movement for your swing, I need to say a little about tight or shortened muscles (lack of flexibility). Tight muscles are the enemy of the sports player! The tighter a muscle is, the smaller range of movement it will have. That will affect not only how well you can move, but may also put abnormal stresses through your joints and cause muscle injury. Most people 'pull' their muscles (muscle strain) or damage ligaments (ligament sprain) when their muscle is at full stretch. If you are more flexible you will be less likely to pull the muscle.

Don't worry – it is never too late to do a little work on your flexibility which will help prevent injury and give you a greater range of movement for your swing. I will talk about how to gain more flexible muscles later, with some simple advice regarding warming up, cooling down and stretches. These don't have to take a long time and can even be done at home. They are very simple but an important part of your routine that will help to keep you playing better and for longer.

I want to make one last point regarding flexibility and age. Thinking of an old person who is bent forward, round-shouldered and head down, just like the road sign that warns of old people crossing – one of the reasons they have become like that is because the muscles and all the soft tissues on the front of their shoulders have shortened as the muscles on their back have weakened. Gravity then pulls them forwards and down. This posture is probably compounded by tightened muscles on the front of their hips. As older people become more sedentary, this can effectively start the process whereby the muscles on the front of their hips begin to become tighter and shorter, adding to the stooped posture. This is an extreme example to illustrate the point, but I want to make sure you understand how muscles can start to tighten without you realising. Much better to work on them now, beginning today, and prevent tightening before it starts.

Not being able to move your joints through their full range of movement will deprive your joint surfaces of their nutrition and can make arthritic changes more likely. This is something none of us want.

How does this affect you as a golfer? Well, without exercise and stretching, your muscles will start to adapt, becoming weaker and tighter which may lead to injury. If you have some shortening around the hips and shoulders, you may find it more difficult to get the backswing and follow through as far as you used to. The range of movement in your left shoulder and your spine will determine the length of your backswing.

You may notice that you are not so good at reaching up for objects... things seem more out of reach than they used to be.

You don't want to allow any of your muscles or soft tissue to get shorter. From this point onwards you could make sure that, with a bit of simple exercising and stretching, you will keep as strong and as supple as possible. The benefits are profound, not only short term, but long term as well. After all, you want to be able to keep playing well for as many years as possible, and still win those games against your arch-rivals at the club!

CHAPTER 3

COMMON GOLF INJURIES AND HOW THEY AFFECT YOUR SWING

Injury is part and parcel of any sport; prevention is the best policy; and if you become injured, with appropriate treatment you will be able to get back to playing soon. However, as we age some changes occur in our bodies. They may be for medical reasons or a side effect from some other issue. Some things we can change with exercise and treatment, and others we can't. My message is, if you can't change it then don't give up! There are ways to modify your technique, modify the equipment you use, or change the way you play so that you can continue playing.

I have heard so many people say, 'I just got too old to play'. What a shame. I bet if we looked at what was stopping them from playing, there may well have been some modifications and/or exercises that could have helped them. I've seen amputees playing golf with their adapted artificial limbs, also people with hip and knee replacements. They have all had to make modifications to their swing, clubs or shoes and work on their conditioning, but they are out there playing... an inspiration to all of us.

Generally speaking, an amateur golf player's injuries are due to:

- Lack of conditioning and coordination

- Lack of technique

- Using too much strength, basically trying too hard

- Jolted swing movements

Lack of conditioning and coordination you already know something about, and the exercises that I give you can address these issues. Exercising will make you stronger, more flexible and coordinated.

The golf swing is a highly technical manoeuvre that requires the player to take his body to the limits of its range of movement in a controlled and coordinated manner. This can be a good thing as it keeps your joints healthier, but a bad thing if it places abnormal and repetitive stresses through the joints, muscles, ligaments and tendons. This is why the stronger and more flexible you are, the better your body is able to cope.

Lack of technique, using too much strength and jolted movements. These can be addressed by your golf Pro and really are essential to work on when taking up golf for the first time. For those already playing, it is well worth some sessions with the Pro followed by practise to improve technique. This is especially worthwhile when you're not under the pressure of a match. After all, nothing ever comes without a bit of perseverance!

I will explain what the common injuries are and what aspect of golf causes them to enable you to look at prevention. This will certainly involve conditioning, good technique and appropriate equipment, but knowing where injuries are most likely to occur will guide you to the areas that you need to work on. Keeping your muscles strong and well balanced will dramatically help prevent injury and pain. You may also have experienced some of these injuries and want to make sure they do not recur.

If you are limited in your movement by chronic pain or a long-standing condition, I'll explain in Chapter 6 how you can compensate for these limitations by adapting your stance, swing or equipment with a little help from your Pro.

This diagram shows how muscles, *tendons* and *ligaments* relate to your bones to help you understand the anatomy of the common injuries.

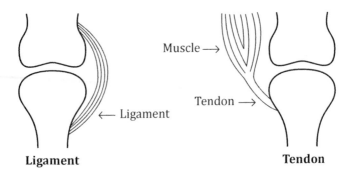

Ligament   **Tendon**

> **Ligaments:** *ligaments are bands of fibrous tissue that join bone to bone or bone to cartilage. They provide support and stability to joints.* **Tendons:** *tendons are tough bands of fibrous tissue that connect muscles to bones. When tendons become inflamed it is called tendonitis.*

> **Sprain***: a sprain is when there is an injury to a ligament.* **Strain***: a strain is when there is an injury to either the muscle or tendon.*

The most common injuries:

Listed below are the most common injuries. If you are experiencing any of these, the description will help you understand why and what may be causing the pain. If you are not, I would still recommend reading about them, as some of the points I make regarding causes will help you think about prevention, if you have a particular weakness or previous condition, before it becomes a problem. All descriptions assume you are a right-handed player. If you are left handed, then the opposite will apply to you.

Later, in Chapters 6 and 7, I will give more detailed advice regarding the treatment and rehabilitation of each injury, and how to adapt in order to continue playing if you have long-standing medical issues and injuries.

Starting from your feet upwards:

Metatarsalgia, or pain in the ball of your foot. This is particularly common in the right foot of the right-handed player and is caused by the extreme pressure put through this joint during both **backswing** and **follow through**.

At the highest point of the **backswing**, up to 90% of your body weight is transferred to your right leg with increased pressure through your toes and heels.

During the **downswing**, 10-20% of your body weight moves towards your left foot, increasing to around 90% by impact.

During the **downswing**, pressure is transferred from your right heel to the ball of your right foot, and during **follow-through**, enormous pressure is put on the ball of your right foot.

Plantar fasciitis is pain under the heel or sometimes along the sole of your foot. The pain is caused when the band of tissue that runs along the sole of your foot, called fascia, becomes inflamed. It can be caused by tightness in your Achilles tendon/calf muscles, ill-fitting shoes, high arches, constant standing/walking (possibly as a result of a change in activity) or weight gain.

The amount of walking involved in golf, the uneven ground, the wearing of ill-fitting golf shoes can all cause plantar fasciitis and it is not uncommon in recreational golfers.

Ankle sprain or 'going over on your ankle'. This means a *sprain* of one or more of the ligaments around your ankle. You hear people saying that they have 'a weak ankle' which basically means that they have sprained one of their ankle ligaments in the past and have not rehabilitated it correctly. This causes the *mechanoreceptors* in their ligaments to not function properly again.

During **impact and follow-through**, your weight is transferred through to your left foot placing stress on the ligaments on the outside of your left ankle.

Walking on uneven ground on the golf course can stress any of your ankle ligaments potentially putting them at risk of injury.

All ligaments and muscles have receptors in them that continually tell the brain how much stretch they are being put under. This allows the brain to automatically correct your posture or movement to prevent over stretching them.

If you sprain your ankle and then do not include any or enough balance and proprioceptive work to stimulate the mechanoreceptors to fire again, the brain never knows when too much stretch is being put through your ankle and so doesn't stop it when it goes too far... hence re-injuring the ankle causing 'a weak ankle'.

> **Mechanoreceptor:** *this is a specialist receptor that responds to mechanical pressure or distortion, e.g. stretch.*

Achilles tendon is the thick tendon on the back of your leg that joins your calf muscles to your heel. It can be partially ruptured or, more seriously, fully ruptured. A lot of people have had a few fibres rupture and have felt a small degree of pain. This can be a troublesome injury, and appropriate treatment and rehabilitation is important to get it back to full function.

Calf muscle injury can seem like an Achilles tendon injury but is located higher up the leg in the muscle belly. This injury tends to occur on the golf course when walking, rather than during the swing. I have heard of golf players injuring their Achilles tendon or calf muscles by slipping on wet and uneven ground, or on slippery wooden bridges over streams.

Knee pain is very common and has many different causes. Sprain of ligaments around the knee can result from trauma, i.e. following falls/slips on uneven ground. Existing medical conditions, i.e. arthritic changes or torn cartilage in the knee, will cause pain and can be exacerbated by the rotational forces put through the knee when playing. The squatting posture adopted by many golfers when picking up the ball or lining up to putt can also cause knee pain.

During **impact**-phase of the swing a vertical compression force of up to 80% of your body weight can be put through your left knee on impact. This can irritate the knee and initiate pain from an existing condition. (Later in the text I mention that less body weight can help prevent/reduce knee pain.)

Hip pain is rarely caused by direct injury to the hip but you could experience pain from an existing hip problem that is exacerbated when attempting a full swing. It is possible to experience a tear of the cartilage in the hip joint due to the increased rotational forces required by the modern swing.

During the **full golf swing**, internal rotation (seen when the knee turns inwards) at the hips is a key movement for an effective swing. Lack of internal rotation will slow the speed of the swing and can cause you to compensate with extra rotation and stress though the spine, cause tightness in your hamstring muscles and predispose you to hamstring injury, back pain and knee pain.

Shoulder pain can be a real problem for a golf player and shoulder problems are often difficult to diagnose. Looking at shoulders is like opening a can of worms! It is a very complicated joint as it can move in so many directions. It consists of many muscles called the 'rotator cuff' that coordinate together to produce the many movements of the arm. If any of these muscles become weaker, it affects the working of the whole rotator cuff. The repetitive movements of golf can cause inflammation of any of the tendons of the rotator cuff, or the pad of fat protecting the shoulder joint may become inflamed if there are any abnormal movements of the shoulder during swing. You will probably need a healthcare professional to diagnose the problem before any treatment can begin. One obvious clue to altered biomechanics of the shoulder is if the levels of your shoulder blades look different. If this is the case, then there is probably a rotator cuff issue. This is an example of when to ask for a professional assessment as treatment will be difficult without some professional guidance.

During the **backswing,** the range of movement in your shoulders determines the length of your backswing. Forcing the club through a longer backswing can put excessive strain on your shoulder joint and initiate pain.

Also during the **backswing**, swinging out too far and keeping your left arm too straight for too long can cause strain on your left shoulder and initiate pain.

At the **top of your backswing**, your left shoulder is in a position that can cause stress on the joint at the back of the shoulder, and stress on the joint at the front of your right shoulder.

During **follow-through,** strain is put on the joint in front of your shoulder (acromio-clavicular joint is the joint between your collar bone and the front of your shoulder), and if you have an excessive follow-through it can initiate pain in this joint.

Any existing arthritic changes around the shoulder area can exacerbate pain if your swing is excessive or jolting in nature.

Golfer's/tennis elbow and wrist pain is caused by inflammation of the tendon (tendonitis) of one of the muscles in the forearm, or wrist, which can be caused by gripping the club too tightly, incorrect grip size, excessive use of the wrist, or hitting the ground causing transmission of the impact force through to your elbow. Lack of technique can cause pain which may result in tendonitis around the wrist, also known as repetitive strain injury. Although often referred to as 'golfer's elbow' (pain on the inside of the elbow), the more common injury experienced by golfers is in fact 'tennis elbow' (pain on the outer side of the elbow).

Your equipment can also be a causative factor of tendonitis and pain. For example, if your golf club shaft is too stiff, it can cause vibrations to be transmitted to your elbow which can result in tendonitis.

Back pain can occur in any region of the spine but different parts are more prone to injury during different phases of the swing. Your lumbar spine (low back), during follow-through, thoracic spine (mid back), site of the pivot point of your swing throughout its duration, and cervical spine (neck), can exhibit pain during downswing with incorrect head movement. Did you know that during a round of golf you could be bending down 30-50 times. Backs don't like bending as it causes repeated stress on the ligaments and discs between the vertebrae. So try to bend your knees rather than your back.

During **follow-through**, hyperextension (arching) of your lower back will cause stress on your lumbar spine (lower back) and can result in pain. This often happens as a compensatory movement if arthritis limits rotation of the hips.

The main regions of the spine

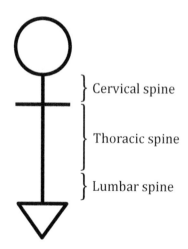

} Cervical spine

} Thoracic spine

} Lumbar spine

Secondary causes of back pain are issues that produce pain in the back, but the actual cause may not be a spinal one. Most can be helped with exercise and/or stretching.

Some examples of secondary pain are:

- **Restarting golf after a break:** as I said earlier, the golf swing takes your spine through a wide arc of movement, from one extreme of rotation on one side through to extreme rotation on the other. Regular play keeps all of the small joints in your spine moving. Excellent! However, if you stop playing golf for a few weeks, maybe because of some other injury, and you are not continuing to take your spine through your normal swing movement during your break, it will begin to stiffen up. When back on the golf course, a degree of back pain can be experienced due to stiffness, This is when a home programme of exercises would prevent this.

- **General lack of rotation of the spine:** some people become stiff over time, or are new to golf and may not be used to taking their spine through such a large arc of movement. Apart from gentle stretching and practise to increase the range of movement, a change in swing may accommodate the lack of rotation and so ease back pain. For this, see Chapter 6.

- **Poor core strength/abdominal weakness:** this is very common, especially in those players who... putting it delicately... have a little more weight around their girth than is ideal. Weak/ stretched abdominal muscles do not support the spine effectively enough and also result in a tipping of the pelvis downwards. This causes the curve in the lumbar spine to become exaggerated, putting strain on the joints and discs in that part of the spine, and resulting in low back pain.

- **Tight quadriceps/hip flexors**: these are the muscles on the front of your thighs and hips. Again, if they are shortened they will pull the pelvis down, causing the increased curve of the lumbar spine as above. Result, low back pain.

- **Tight hamstrings:** this is very common as not many people regularly stretch their hamstrings so they can become tight/shortened. This will also tilt the pelvis and produce stress on the spine.

I hope this doesn't sound all doom and gloom! Golf can keep you fit and healthy, but you need to be aware of some of the stresses it can put on your body so that you can avoid them becoming a problem.

The Chartered Society of Physiotherapy has produced a series of advice leaflets, in conjunction with Arthritis Research UK, for use by the general public. They are designed to give advice on what exercises can help manage and treat common conditions. The web link is: www.csp.org.uk/publications/exercise-advice-leaflets. These leaflets cover foot pain, carpal tunnel syndrome, knee pain, neck pain, shoulder pain, back pain and tennis elbow.

CHAPTER 4

SIMPLE INJURY PREVENTION

This is one of the most important aspects of your sporting life and something that you can have some control over. Some injuries are unavoidable and are part and parcel of playing sport, but there are many that you can prevent.

Simple actions you can take to help avoid injury

Prevention is better than cure, not only because you don't want to miss your golf, but also because each time an injury occurs, your body lays down scar tissue to repair it. This scar tissue can cause secondary issues of movement and may be a site for re-injury, especially if not treated correctly following initial injury.

There are some very simple steps that you can take to help prevent injury whilst playing. This is important as it can be frustrating to miss out while your friends play.

It is also important to understand that there is a little work involved to prevent injury. Poor conditioning of the body and poor technique will cause most injuries. Having worked as a physiotherapist for more than 30 years, I know doing exercises is boring. If they are too complicated, they won't get done, and only the very highly motivated can stick to a demanding programme... we'd all just rather be out there playing than exercising. However, good body conditioning is the best way to keep you healthy and fit to play.

The technique advice I leave to the golf Pros. If you have an existing condition that limits your play, or swing, there are some equipment adaptations/additions that, together with advice from your Pro, may allow you to find a way to work around them. I give examples of this in Chapter 6.

What else can you do to prevent injury or pain?

- Knee pain can be helped by **appropriate footwear,** with the appropriate **support inside** the shoes, and possibly a change in studs.

- Golfer's elbow and some shoulder problems can be prevented by a proper **assessment of your swing and your clubs**, including grip size.

- Did you know that you need to be **properly hydrated** to prevent muscle fatigue which can cause injury? Golf is a long game, and the older we get the easier it is to become dehydrated.

- Appropriate **clothing to maintain core temperature** will help the circulation to your hands and feet. Technical clothing is great for this.

- Possibly most important of all is **warming up** before play and **cooling down** after.

- Avoidance of **pain and fatigue** which will affect your performance, compromise your swing and might predispose you to injury.

(If you have any existing health issues then advice from your GP may be needed to ensure that you can play to your full potential within the limits of your medical condition.)

Footwear

Most players go to the golf shop and buy golf shoes. That's great, but not all golf shoes offer moulded insoles that totally support your feet. If you tend to over pronate your feet (see diagram on page 59), without suitable support, this can have a detrimental effect on your knees and to a lesser extent on your hips and can result in pain.

Our feet are designed to rotate inwards slightly as we land on our heels and transmit the motion forwards through our feet. This small amount of pronation (inward rotation) acts as a sort of shock absorber.

However, some of us tend to over rotate and our ankles lean inwards when we weight bear through our feet.

Our feet are made up of many bones, each joined by ligaments, with many muscles around the foot (either in our foot or coming from our leg attaching to the bones in the foot). The differing pull of the muscles can cause the foot to be distorted in many directions if the forces on it are great enough. Pronation is caused either when there is an uneven pull on the bones around the heel or it is due to developing flat feet. Flat feet are caused by the arches dropping and the feet rotating inwards, again pronation. Most of us don't realise when this is the case, but biomechanically it spells problems for the knees. It is gradual, and unless you are specifically looking you probably wouldn't notice it. If you have some knee pain, it is worth looking at your feet! This is because, as the foot rolls in, the joint around the heel rotates and this puts stress directly onto the ankles and knees. Without any form of correction this will continue and predispose the ankles and knees to pain and abnormal wear and tear on the joint surfaces, better known as arthritic changes.

Diagram showing over-pronation at the ankle

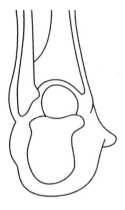 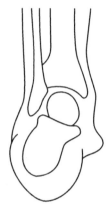

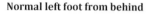

Normal left foot from behind   **Over-pronated left foot**

So what can you do? My advice, if you have over-pronating feet, is to buy a decent pair of orthotic insoles and replace the insoles in your golf shoes with these. The insole should give good support to your arches and around your heel bone (calcaneus) to prevent it rotating.

I over pronate my feet and have insoles in most of my shoes as I take the view that I always want to keep my feet properly aligned. However, a podiatrist did explain to me that while insoles are very good at keeping your feet supported and well aligned, if you wear them all of the time then the muscles in your feet can get weaker. So, it is a good idea to walk around in bare feet, or in shoes without the insoles, for short periods each day to exercise your feet. I walk around at home either in bare feet or my beloved slippers (with no insoles!) and have the shoes with insoles for when I go out.

If I feel that there isn't enough shock absorbency in the heel of the insole, I buy a gel pad and stick it in the heel area. Gel pads are available in all pharmacies and large supermarkets. They are sold for easing pressure on feet when wearing high heeled shoes but I have found them just as good for my trainers. The gel pads act as a shock absorber when put in the heel area and take away some of the pressure as my heel hits the ground during walking or running. This has helped protect my knees from increased pressure on my joint surfaces. You may want to play around with different insoles, with and without shock absorbers, to see what is best for you. Some insoles have built-in gel pads.

Good insoles can be found in some pharmacies, some sports shops, particularly running shops, golf/tennis shops and on-line. If you have concerns or more complicated issues with your feet, an orthotist (healthcare professional trained to assess for orthotic appliances such as splints, braces and special footwear), podiatrist (healthcare professional trained to deal with problems of the feet) or physiotherapist should be able to help you. Any of these professionals can prescribe custom-made insoles to specifically fit your feet. If you do want to see a physiotherapist, orthotist or podiatrist, only use ones that are registered with the HCPC (Health and Care Professions Council). You can check this on line at www.hpc-uk.org

You can also look up flat feet, causes and treatment, on the NHS Choices website (www.nhs.uk).

The professional body for chiropodists and podiatrists also have information on their website at: www.scpod.org

The professional body for orthotists is found at: www.bapo.com

Golf studs

Golf studs are definitely worth a mention. They are designed to prevent your foot slipping during the golf swing, but this in itself can cause problems. If you have knee or hip pain, it may be that the studs are preventing some of the rotation of your leg through the swing and therefore putting abnormally high pressure through your knee and/or hip. If you suffer from any pain in the ball of your foot, studs can be contributing to the pain. This is often due to the positioning of the studs channelling the pressure to that exact point on your foot.

In either case, I would recommend trying to re-position your studs, use softer studs or try without them to see how it affects your pain. You can also try 'trainer specific' golf shoes with rubberised soles that will absorb some of the impact travelling up through your feet. You could speak to the golf Pro, a specialist in a golf shop and/or one of the healthcare professionals listed above if you continue to have problems playing with studs.

Assessment of your swing and clubs

When assessing the golf swing, one of the biggest equipment issues that struck me was, why do most amateur players use standard golf clubs? The majority of players that I interviewed played with either male or female standard size clubs. I found this surprising as we don't come in standard sizes. If you are playing with standard clubs, you have to adapt your body to fit the club. This may not be such an issue with young, adaptable bodies, but the older we get the less adaptable we are. So ill-fitting clubs can make it much harder to achieve a good swing technically and can predispose your body to injury. An assessment in a golf shop, or by your Pro, may just make all the difference. It may be a simple change to longer/shorter shafts, or clubs with a bit more flex.

A player I met had chosen her clubs because of their colour, and as beautiful as they were, they were not the ones the technician had advised her to get. Of course, it is a personal choice, but I would urge you to think carefully when choosing your clubs. You know what is important for you and for your game. I appreciate that specifically prescribed clubs may cost more, but what price would you put on protecting your body?

I would also recommend experimenting with the grip size of your clubs if you are experiencing any pain in your elbow or wrist. The smaller the grip, the harder your muscles have to work to grip it. Changing the grip size will help redirect some of the forces to different parts of your tendons, allow your hands to grip a little less forcibly and so ease the tension on the tendons.

(NB Too thin a grip causes too much hand action in the swing, too thick a grip resists hand action.)

Hydration/dehydration

This is one of the most commonly overlooked health aspects of the amateur sports player. Hydration, or preventing dehydration, is very important for your body, not just when you are playing golf but every day. Your body is made up of at least half water, and water is vital for your body to function efficiently. Whilst playing any sport, becoming dehydrated will affect your muscles causing them to fatigue more quickly and so predispose you to injury.

The European Food Safety Authority (quoted on the NHS Choices website listed below), recommends that women drink around 1.6 litres of fluid, and men around 2.0 litres of fluid a day. The more active you are, the more fluid you will need. The NHS Choices website (www.nhs. uk/conditions/Dehydration/Pages/Introduction.aspx) recommends that:

- For any exercise that lasts longer than 30 minutes, drink fluid while you are doing it. The more you sweat the more you will need to drink.

- Water is usually enough for low intensity exercise up to 50 minutes.

- For higher intensity exercise, lasting more than 50 minutes, or lower intensity exercise lasting hours, a sports drink would be of benefit.

This is just a guideline, and you should know that as we age, our bodies can dehydrate at a faster rate and our thirst levels can drop. So we may not always realise we are becoming dehydrated.

A vascular surgeon (doctor who specialises in the blood vessels of your body) gave a talk in my area and said that the three main risks to an individual's vascular systems were smoking, obesity and dehydration. Wow! I hadn't appreciated exactly how important good hydration was, and apparently a lot of us may often be dehydrated, to a degree, and not know it. Add exercising to that and you can see how important it is to manage your fluid intake, especially when playing sport! So, ensure you drink enough when you play golf.

If you have any medical issues with calories or diabetes or you are unsure what drink is best for you to maintain your hydration levels, then I would recommend asking your GP for advice on what will be best, given your medical history.

Clothing to maintain core temperature

One of the effects of ageing is that the circulation in your extremities is less efficient. In cold weather your body compounds this by trying to keep your core warm at the expense of your extremities. By layering up correctly, your core stays warm enabling your body to keep your extremities warmer. Wearing the right gear for the conditions will keep you warm and help your muscles work more efficiently.

Ideally, your first layer will be a wicking textile, so not cotton. If you sweat at all, cotton will become damp and lose its insulating effects causing you to lose heat. Wear a synthetic, breathable layer to draw the sweat away. Your second layer should be an insulating layer, e.g. a fleece, and if you need a third layer then a loose, waterproof and windproof-material top or jacket would be good. That's the theory. If it does not allow you enough movement, then I would recommend layering down for your shot and then re-layering before your core temperature drops.

Warming up and cooling down

Many recreational golf players do not warm up adequately before they play which immediately predisposes them to injury, and the older you get the more easily this will happen. We need to warm our muscles up in order to increase the blood flow, make the contraction and relaxation of the muscle more efficient and give the muscle and joints the nutrients and fuel they need. Mental preparation, before playing a game, is also an important part of a warming up routine. It prepares you for your sport and stimulates the neural pathways (connections between the muscles and the brain) which help to produce a better quality of swing, thus helping you begin the game with better technique. Why not start as you mean to go on?

Most people feel a bit awkward warming up in front of others, especially if they are the only one doing it. So, warm up at home beforehand. If you do a good enough warm up, the effects can last for up to 40 minutes. Hopefully that will be plenty of time for you to get to the club and start playing with pre-warmed muscles.

Cooling down after is also important as it gives you the opportunity to gently stretch your muscles. This helps maintain their flexibility which is so important to maintain that swing. Again, it will not take long and is well worth the few minutes to prevent injuries in the future.

A little note on flexibility... we could all probably do with being a little more flexible in certain muscles. Unless you take your joints through their full range of movement regularly, they will begin to adapt and shorten. In fact, it is not only your muscles but all of the connective tissue, ligaments, tendons (collectively called soft tissue), that can shorten. A 75 year old that I play tennis with asked me one day, 'Why are my legs getting longer?' by which he meant that he was finding it difficult to reach his feet. This immediately told me that he was losing some of his flexibility, and so I talked to him about a stretching programme. A few months later it appeared that his legs had stopped getting longer!

Biomechanically, our bodies are set up to work in the most efficient way, and if any joint can't move through its full range due to shortening of the soft tissue, then it will affect the movement of that joint. Needless to say, it will also affect how well we perform any movement involving that joint, and it may impact our swing.

Another really good reason to take our joints through their full range of movement is to give the joint surface the nutrition it needs. The cartilage (a protective layer of tissue that lines each joint surface) requires nutrition from the fluid in the joints to keep it healthy. The fluid reaches all parts of the cartilage by the joint being moved through its range. If an area is deprived of nutrition, then it will start to degrade and this can be the start of arthritic change which is to some extent avoidable.

Most injuries to muscles occur when they are at full stretch. If your muscles are tight, then that will occur sooner in the movement. A flexible muscle will adapt to the length required of it most of the time. Even professional athletes can't avoid the occasional muscle strain, pulled hamstring, etc. Generally they don't because they work to maintain their muscles to achieve the appropriate length for their sport.

A word to the wise: you should never stretch a cold muscle as this can lead to muscle damage more easily. It is much safer to stretch a warm muscle.

Pain and fatigue

Pain and fatigue cause our brains to slow down in understanding where our body is in space and where our joints are in space. This is called proprioception, or joint position sense, as described earlier.

Proprioception is vital for the sports person and directly affects skill level. When you become tired your joint position sense decreases, and this can cause skill level to drop and injuries to occur, especially during the golf swing, when your brain needs to know exactly where your body is in space to produce a fluid, balanced movement.

Existing medical conditions

If you have any sort of existing medical problems that may be affected by exercise or any of these issues, or if you are in any doubt as to what is right and safe for you to do, then you should speak to your GP or see a suitable healthcare professional who can specifically advise you.

Arthritis and pain/injury

One last comment regarding arthritis... I have been asked, 'If I do more exercise, am I wearing my joints out sooner? Will arthritis become worse or start sooner?'

As far as arthritis goes, correctly exercising the muscles helps to keep them strong enough to support your joints. It also helps to keep the joint surfaces nourished. Both of these outcomes help prevent arthritic changes and pain from occurring and so help to keep your joints younger. An excellent reason, therefore, to get on with those exercises!

An orthopaedic consultant told me of a study carried out in America which looked at the effects of exercise on the knee joint of adults who regularly exercised compared to adults who lived a more sedentary lifestyle. It found that exercise had no detrimental effect overall on the joints compared to not exercising. Plus there were all of the additional health benefits of exercise. So, you probably don't 'wear out' your joints more quickly by exercising them, particularly if you have a balanced exercise programme... good news for all of us. After all, you are playing to stay healthy as well as staying healthy to play.

CHAPTER 5

HOME EXERCISE PROGRAMME TO KEEP YOU FIT FOR GOLF

This is the section that I get really excited about... if you do this right then you may never have to look at the treatment section as I hope you will avoid some of the injuries and be able to carry on playing for many years to come!

This is 'the what and the how', a small group of exercises I have chosen that will work the main muscle groups. There are many different exercises that you can do to achieve the same outcome, but these are my suggestions to strengthen you with minimal disruption to your life. Plus, they work on the main muscle groups that are important for your golf, working the muscles symmetrically and so preventing muscle imbalance.

If you want a more demanding exercise programme you could join a gym. For those who want to be stronger for longer, have younger muscles and be able to prevent those injuries by exercising at home, this chapter tells you what you need to do.

How could you have a set of exercises that you are happy to work through and don't get bored doing? The answer is to include them in your everyday life... make them part of your everyday activities. That's not to say that you have to do them every day – usually three times a week is enough to increase and then maintain strength.

There are some simple exercises that you can do at home whilst sitting watching TV, standing when washing up at the sink, when you go up/down your stairs and even when you are brushing your teeth. I will explain each exercise in detail with a corresponding picture and why it is important to your golf performance.

Some exercises are really simple and part of what you already do each day. For example, when you are going up stairs, go up two at a time and slowly. This works your thigh and bottom muscles more (quads and gluts), the resistance being your body weight. When you are sitting watching TV, hold a bottle of water or small weight (described below), and you can effectively exercise your arm muscles as you watch. The resistance is provided by the weight of the water. There are countless exercises for the legs, arms and body that you can do sitting down with a length of stretchy band, or weights, to give you the resistance to build your muscles. My favourite example of an everyday exercise is, when brushing your teeth, always stand on one leg. You will be stimulating your balance mechanisms. Balance is an essential skill that needs to be worked on to maintain, but is easy to forget.

What equipment will you need apart from a TV to watch? You will need a chair and something to act as a balance/support when exercising on just one leg. You will need stairs or a step, a bottle of water, and some weights or a couple of lengths of elastic resistive bands. I explain what these are and how to use them later in this chapter, and in Chapter 9 where you can buy them. If you are using resistive bands, then you will probably need a couple as you will find that you need a stronger one for your leg muscles and an easier one for your arm muscles.

If you do not want to use the bands, then you can use some form of weights. These can be purchased from most sport shops or online and some supermarkets also sell exercise weights. Or you can make your own weights by using a filled water bottle for some exercises though I suspect that it won't be heavy enough for most of them. Ankle weights are particularly useful as you can use them in your hands as well as a resistance for your legs. I have included examples of exercises that you can do using either the bands or weights.

Each piece of equipment that requires purchasing should cost less than a good bottle of wine.

How often should you do the exercises?

If you are going to do the exercises at a set time in your day, then you need to do them at least three times a week. If you are going to incorporate them into your daily activities then great, you are doing them daily. Obviously, the more you do the better the results and the quicker you will be able to progress them. When you have done the exercises for about eight weeks you will then be at your maintenance level. The more you have managed to increase your resistance and number of exercises over that time, the stronger your muscles will be. So you will be maintaining stronger muscles and that can only be a good thing.

You don't have to stop increasing the resistance or number of exercises you do at the end of eight weeks, you can continue to increase them if you want. It would be nice to think that you have got yourself as strong as you are happy with.

Some **golden rules** regarding any exercise programme that you need to be aware of:

- If you experience any pain then stop. Do not work through pain. You need to find out the cause of the pain and treat it accordingly.

- Always have a stable base when doing an exercise otherwise your muscle tension will increase when trying to balance and this can cause injury. Obviously the balance exercises are the exception, but even then you must be able to reach to hold on to a stable object in case you start to over-balance and need to right yourself.

- You must exercise regularly to gain any benefit, so the best programme is an ongoing one. The shorter the time you have been exercising, the quicker you will lose any gains you have made if you stop. If you have been exercising regularly for a long time, then you will be able to occasionally skip some sessions without much, if any, loss of muscle strength. Great! You don't have to do them when you go on holiday!

- Don't over-do it. Rest is also important as this allows the changes in your muscles to occur.

- Always start each exercise gently to act as a warm up. Ideally do the movement first a few times without the resistance to warm your muscles before making them work harder. Gradually build up how hard you are working with each repetition of the exercise.

- When using a resistive band or weights, ensure that you have read the manufacturer's safety precautions, guidelines and care of equipment before use.

- It takes 6-8 weeks for the muscles and nervous systems to adapt to your new exercises and so you will not notice great changes before then.

- If you have any existing medical conditions or ailments that you know of that may be affected by the exercises, then I would advise that you check them out with your GP or physiotherapist to ensure that they are suitable for your condition as they may need some adaptions.

You want to increase the strength of your muscles through the whole of the range of movement, so always try to take the band or weight through the whole movement.

I include doing the exercises on both sides of your body, not just your dominant side. This is because it is really important to try to get symmetry of muscle strength in your body. I have already mentioned the term 'muscle imbalance' which is basically one side being stronger than the other. This can happen to regular golf players and cause abnormal pulling on your body. Muscle imbalance leads to abnormal stresses on your joints. So let's keep symmetrical with the exercises.

I have included a section with specific exercises to strengthen hamstring and hip muscle groups. I have included these as 'extra' exercises for those who wish to work specifically on these muscles because of injury or weakness.

Most exercise programmes are made up of what we call 'sets and reps'. Sets mean the number of times you do the group of reps. Reps mean the number of repetitions, or times, you do the exercise. For example, bending your arm 10 reps for 3 sets means... bend your arm 10 times, rest then do it again 10 times, rest and repeat again. You have done 10 bends 3 times, so 10 reps, 3 sets... 30 bends in total.

Once you start exercising you'll find out how easy it is and be surprised at how soon you start increasing your sets and reps as you get stronger. I will explain in more detail later how sets and reps work and how to increase them.

I have included tables in Chapter 8 that you can copy and use to keep track of how many sets and reps for each exercise you are doing and with what band or weight. By six weeks you'll be able to see your progression, so you will know you're getting stronger and that you're building up those muscle fibres!

How will I know it is having an effect?

There are several ways you can measure that your exercise regime is working:

1. You are increasing your sets and reps.

2. You are increasing the resistance of your band or the weight you are using.

3. The length of time you can balance on one leg with eyes open and then with eyes closed is increasing.

4. You will feel it when playing golf. Your swing may well feel more controlled as your balance, body awareness and muscle reaction times improve as they get stronger.

5. You are staying fitter, with fewer injuries than your friends. This will be much more noticeable in the long term.

6. You could try to measure the girth of your legs or arms, but realistically you would have to really 'bulk' up your muscle to do this. Also, you may be losing stored body fat as a result of the exercises, so you may experience no change as you gain muscle but lose fat.

Sets and Reps

If you attend a gym with a personal trainer, they will devise an exercise programme for you that is based on 'sets and reps'. It is a way to count and increase each exercise in a more regulated fashion. If you want to increase the exercises as the professionals do, then you can use sets and reps as described below. If you would rather just gradually increase the number of times you do the exercise instead of grouping them in sets and reps, that's fine. Just make a note of the number of times you do the exercise. Do whatever works best for you so long as you try to slowly increase the number and resistance over an 8-week period.

When you start your exercise programme, you should start gently. Increase as you begin to find the exercise easy to do. You don't want to rush it and risk injury by increasing too quickly. Decide what is right for you so that you feel you have done a bit of work but not tired yourself out. Remember, it takes about 6-8 weeks for your muscles and nerves to fully adapt, but hopefully by the time you reach 6-8 weeks you will have increased to a level that you can continue with as a maintenance programme, i.e. you don't have to increase the amount of reps, sets or weights anymore as you have reached the strength that you are happy with.

If you want to use sets and reps to count your exercises, then start with:

One set of 5-10 reps of each exercise; then once you have increased to 10 reps change to:

Two sets of 5-10 reps of each exercise; and once you have increased to 10 reps change to:

Three sets of 10 reps of each exercise and increase to 15 reps.

Once you are at this level of three sets of 15 reps, you may want to increase the resistance and start again. You can do this by getting a more resistive band, doubling up the band, or increasing the weight you are lifting. Or you may want to keep increasing the number of sets that you do... whatever works for you. Try not to get too carried away as it will take too long to get through the exercises and you will get bored. After 6-8 weeks when you are working at maintenance rather than strengthening, you shouldn't need to increase the resistance unless you want to. Some people are more enthusiastic than others, but do keep at it, remembering that you are investing in your future, and if you don't use it you will lose it!

Photographs of exercises and stretches

These are my suggestions for the sort of exercises that you can to do at home. Have a go, and you'll see how easy they are, and you can do most of them whilst doing your usual activities. I have grouped them together depending on what muscles they are strengthening. Ideally you should do all of them, but if you feel that is too much for you, then I suggest as a minimum do all 3 of the back and hip flexibility exercises (perhaps in bed before getting up in the morning) to maintain your range of movement, and one from each group of the strengthening exercises. The aim is to try to fit them into some of the things that you do each day, e.g. when standing at the sink, try to do the heel off the floor exercise (exercise to strengthen calf muscles), when getting out of a chair, do it a couple of times (exercise 3 to strengthen knee and hip muscles), do the step ups each time you go up the stairs (exercise 5 to strengthen knee and hip muscles). Changing a few little things now can help keep your muscles stronger.

Start with a low number of reps and gradually build them up. It will help if you keep a rough note of where you are with them. My test group of golfers doing the exercises said that after a couple of weeks they soon became routine. They were still enjoying the challenge, particularly balancing whilst doing various activities, climbing stairs two at a time and lifting their heels up even when standing in a supermarket queue! After a few weeks they realised how much they had progressed and felt stronger for it... excellent! When you keep at it and progress you'll have the satisfaction of knowing you are doing something very positive and investing in your future, and that's a great motivator in itself.

Don't forget to read any safety instructions and precautions that come with the equipment you buy. Make sure you are wearing suitable footwear and clothing, and then you're ready to get started and enjoy yourself!

EXERCISES FOR HIP AND BACK FLEXIBILITY

These exercises help to maintain the flexibility of your hips and lower back needed for the rotation during your swing.

Exercise 1

Lying on your back with both knees bent up and feet flat on the bed, gently take both knees to one side, as far as is comfortable, and then take to the other side. Repeat five times to each side.

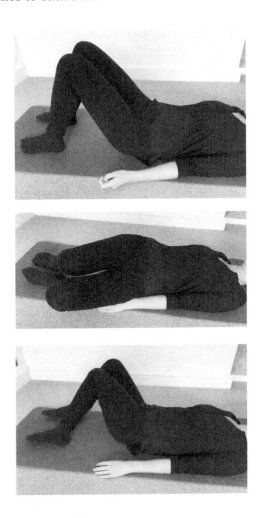

Exercise 2

Lying on your back with both knees bent up and feet flat on the bed, gently push your lower back into the bed and then gently arch it up. Repeat five times.

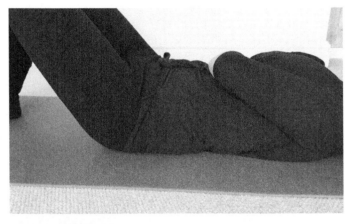

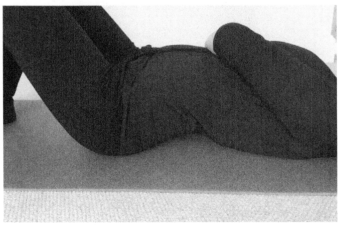

Exercise 3

Lying on your back, keep both legs straight, then roll both legs inwards so that your knees are facing each other and then roll them outwards so that both knees point outwards.

This exercise helps to maintain rotation at your hips and helps stretch out the muscles on the front of your hips.

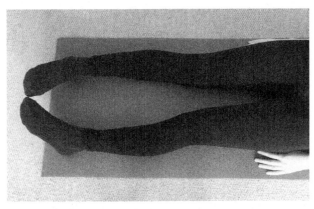

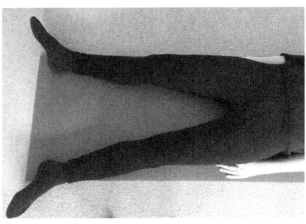

EXERCISES TO STRENGTHEN YOUR WRIST AND FOREARM MUSCLES

These exercises help to strengthen the wrist muscles for better wrist control through the swing.

Fill a small bottle (500cl) with water or hold a small weight. Your arm should be resting on the arm of a chair, or along a table edge, with just your wrist hanging over the end, palm facing downwards.

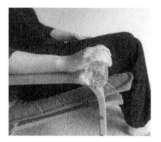 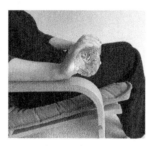

Lift the bottle by only bending your wrist up; do not lift your arm up off of the support/table. Hold for a count of five then relax. Then with your wrist cocked up as before, move your hand from side to side, five times each way, then relax.

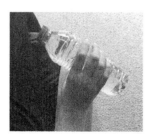 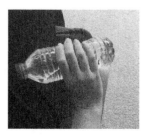

EXERCISES TO STRENGTHEN SHOULDERS AND UPPER BACK MUSCLES

These exercises strengthen the shoulder and upper back muscles which produce control and speed of the golf club. Exercise 3 particularly strengthens the lats which provide control in the back swing and power during the downswing.

Exercise 1

Hold the band in each hand securely, with arms straight out in front of you, pull the band apart as far as you can, hold for a count of five and then relax. This strengthens your back and shoulder muscles.

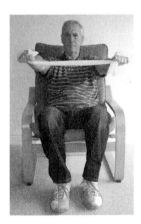 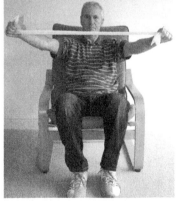

The shorter the length of band you pull, the greater the resistance. You could also progress by tying one end to form a loop and effectively doubling the band. Ensure that you hold the band tightly and any knot is secure.

Exercise 2

As in no.1 but lift the band above your head, arms straight and pull apart. Hold for count of five then relax. Again, this strengthens your back and shoulder muscles.

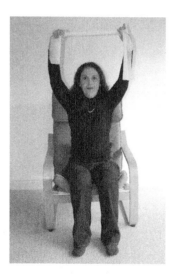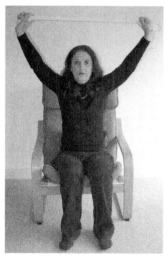

The shorter the band, the harder the resistance. Again, you could progress by tying one end to form a loop and effectively doubling the band. You must ensure that the knot is secure to prevent it coming undone.

Exercise 3

This exercise strengthens the lats which provide control in the back swing and power during the downswing.

Loop the band over the top of a door and place a chair just in front of the door. Sitting with your back to the door, wedge the chair against the door so it doesn't move. (Check that the top of the door is smooth so that it does not damage your band. If you put a small towel on the top of the door, it will protect the band and help to stop it slipping off the door). Take the ends of the band in each hand and slowly pull the band downwards until your arms are straight. Hold for a count of five and then relax.

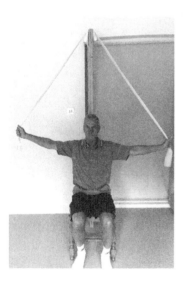 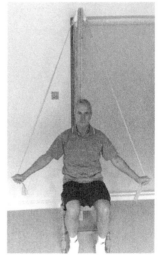

EXERCISE TO STRENGTHEN THE ROTATIONAL MUSCLES IN YOUR BODY

This exercise strengthens your oblique muscles which are important for balance and controlled rotation of the body, particularly during downswing.

Exercise to the left:

Place one end of the band securely under your right thigh near your knee; hold the other end with your left hand. Diagonally stretch the band until your arm is straight and the band is at about a 45 degree angle rotating your body to the left as far as is comfortable. Hold for a count of five then relax. The shorter the band, the greater the resistance, so you need to hold it so that you feel your muscles are working.

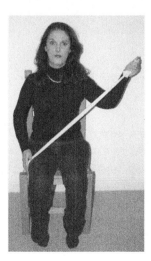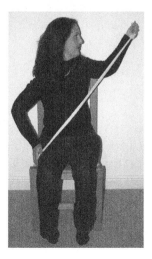

Exercise to the right:

Repeat as above but with the band under your left thigh and stretch the band with your right arm.

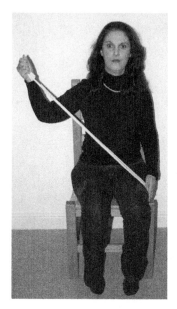 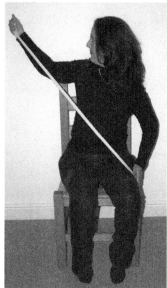

EXERCISES TO STRENGTHEN HIP AND KNEE MUSCLES

These exercises strengthen the hips and knees which are important for balance and power to the swing, particularly during backswing and downswing. This also helps to maintain balance at the end of the swing.

Exercise 1

Tie the band into a loop and place around your knees. Place your feet apart so that you feel tension in the band. Keeping your knees apart, slowly stand up. Do not let your knees drop inwards.

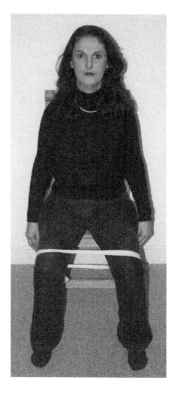
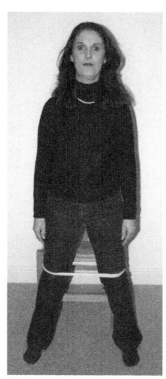

Exercise 2

This exercise is called the single leg dip. Stand so that you can hold onto something secure (back of heavy chair/ table top). Stand on just your right leg and maintain your balance by holding on to the chair. Gently bend your right knee and then slowly straighten. Ensure that you don't let your left hip drop when you are standing on your right leg as this will help keep your pelvis level.

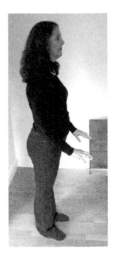 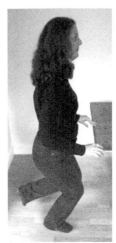 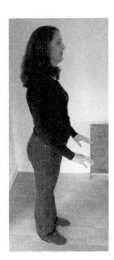

Don't let your knee fall inwards. This is important so that you exercise the correct muscles. Repeat with the other leg.

Exercise 3

Whenever you get up from a chair during the day, try to get up slowly and get up/sit down a couple of times before actually leaving the chair. Do not use your hands to help you stand. This will work all of your leg muscles.

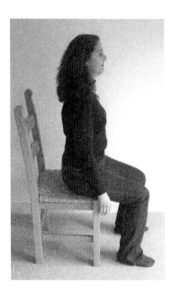 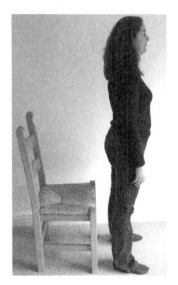

Exercise 4

Walk up your stairs slowly two at a time; hold on to the banister for balance if needed.

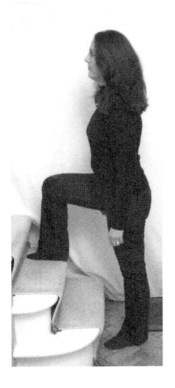 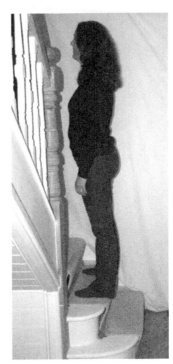

Exercise 5

Each time you go upstairs, place your right foot on the bottom step. Step up and down with the left foot, keeping the right foot on the step all the time. Make sure that you keep your right knee in line – do not let it fall inwards. Do this exercise 10 times then change feet. The first 10 step-ups you are working your right quads, gluts and hamstrings. When you swap feet you'll work the other side and it only takes a minute!

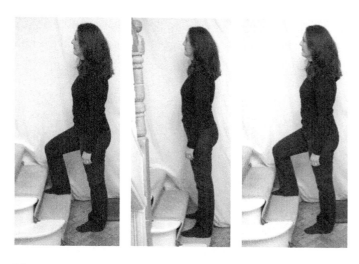

If you want to progress this exercise, you can do it holding some small weights in your hands to increase the resistance on your legs

EXERCISE TO STRENGTHEN THE CALF MUSCLES

This exercise strengthens the calf muscles which are important for balance and transferring your weight forward onto your toes.

Stand facing a support, gently lift your heels off the ground so that you are standing on tip toe and then lower back down. You can get into the habit of doing this whenever you are standing at the sink doing the washing up. Always have a stable base or a stable object you can hold on to if you start to lose your balance when doing standing exercises.

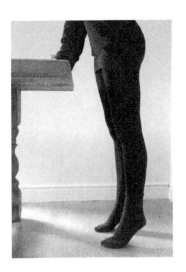
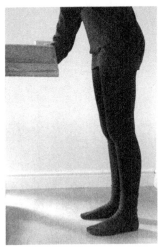

EXERCISES TO IMPROVE BALANCE

These exercises improve your balance which is essential for control throughout the swing from addressing the ball to the finish of the follow-through.

Exercise 1

When brushing your teeth, try to get into the habit of balancing on one leg and then the other. You may have to hold on to something at first, but gradually your balance should improve and you won't have to.

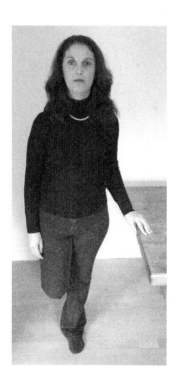

Exercise 2

See how long you can balance on one leg first with your eyes open and then with them closed. It is really hard to do with the eyes closed, but if you can improve the length of time you do it, you will know that you really are improving your muscle power, coordination and consequently your balance.

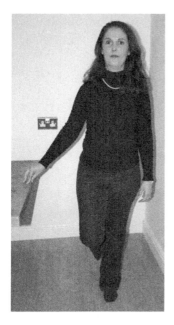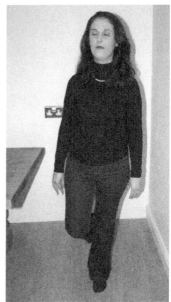

ADVANCED EXERCISES THAT STRENGTHEN ALL MUSCLE GROUPS AT THE SAME TIME

These exercises strengthen all of the muscle groups that are needed to produce a smooth and efficient swing.

With a long piece of band (at least 3m), stand holding the ends in your hands and place your feet shoulder width apart on the band. Bend both knees as if you are addressing the golf ball. Hold your tummy in and keep your head looking forwards.

Keeping arms straight, lift both arms up to 90 degrees so that they are perpendicular to the floor. Hold for a count of five and then relax. Gradually build up number of repetitions.

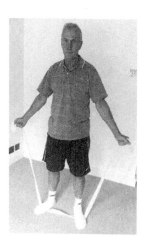 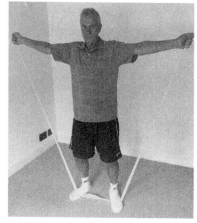

As above, but when your arms are at 90 degrees (hands at level of your shoulders), keep your arms straight and rotate/twist your body from one side to the other, keeping your arms in line with your body.

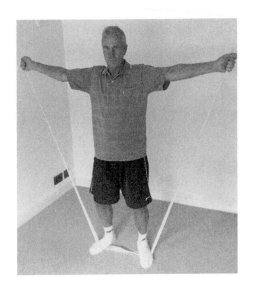

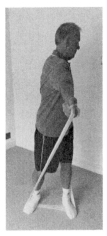 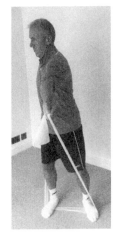

EXTRA EXERCISES FOR THOSE WHO WANT TO SPECIFICALLY EXERCISE THEIR HAMSTRINGS, HIP ABDUCTORS AND GLUTEAL MUSCLE GROUPS

I have included these exercises as 'extras' as they are intended for those players who have a specific weakness which is affecting their swing or who are recovering from a specific injury.

Some are easier than others so it is best to start with the easier ones and move on to the harder ones when the muscles are stronger. Always check with your GP or healthcare professional if you are unsure which exercise is best for your specific weakness.

Lying on your back, hip strengthening with weights (lying on your back makes it easier for muscles)

Lying down with a weight on your ankle, keep your leg straight and take it out to the side by about 30 cm (12 inches), hold it there for count of five then bring back to starting position slowly. Repeat with each leg as per your sets and reps level. This exercise will strengthen the muscle around your hip.

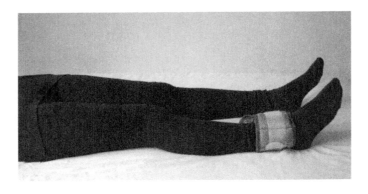

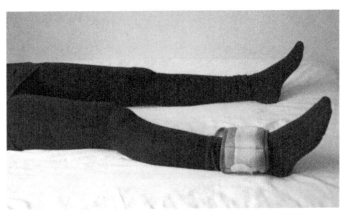

Lying on your side, hip and gluts strengthening with weights (harder work for muscles)

Lie on your side with the ankle weight securely fixed around your ankle. Lift your leg straight up, about 30 cm (12 inches) above your other leg. Do not bend your knee or your hip. Hold for a count of five then relax. Repeat as per your sets and reps level. Repeat with the other leg.

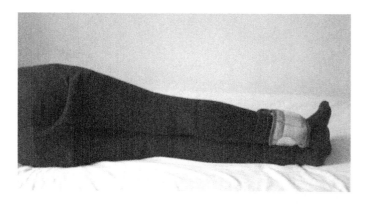

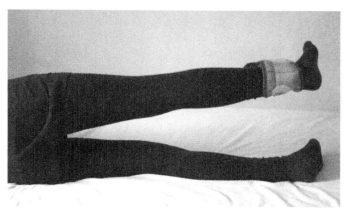

Lying on your back, hip strengthening with a band (easier work for muscles)

Tie the band securely into a loop around your ankles. Lying on your back, slowly pull your feet apart until you feel the muscles around your hips working. Hold for a count of five and then relax. Repeat as per your reps and sets level.

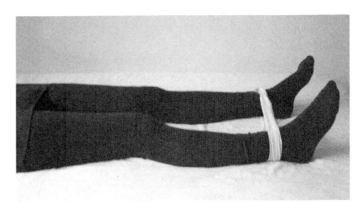

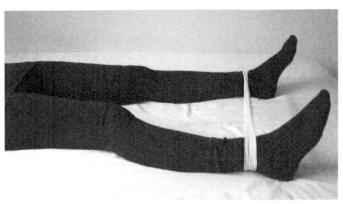

Lying on your side, hip and gluts strengthening with a band (harder work for muscles)

Tie the band in a secure loop and place around your ankles. Lie on your side. Keep your knee and hip straight. Slowly lift your upper leg up, keeping your knee straight until you feel the muscles around your hips working. Hold for a count of five then lower back down slowly. Repeat as per your sets and reps level. Repeat with your other leg by lying on your other side.

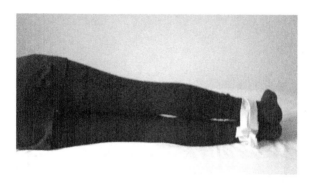

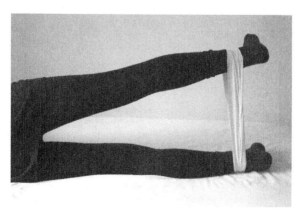

Lying on your front, hamstrings strengthening with weights

Lie on your tummy with the weight around your ankle. Slowly bend your knee keeping it in a straight line, i.e. not letting it wobble side to side. Bend it up to about 90 degrees and then lower back down slowly. Repeat as your reps and sets level. Repeat with the other leg.

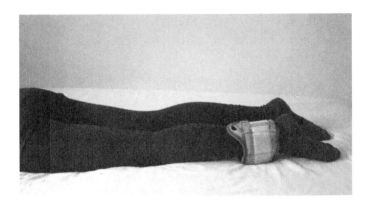

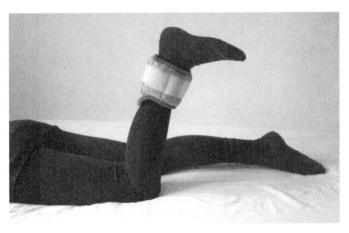

STRETCHES

Stretches are important to maintain the flexibility of your muscle, ligaments and tendons. You should try to get into the habit of stretching within 10 minutes of when you finish your golf. You can also do stretches after an exercise session if you are keen. The more regularly you do stretches, the more effective they will be. You should only stretch your muscles when they are warmed up; stretching on cold muscles can cause damage and muscle tears.

Stretches should be done in a comfortable, stable position. After you start the stretch, continue until you feel tension. Hold it there for about 30 seconds then relax. Do not bounce through the stretch, and ensure you breathe normally. Ideally repeat each stretch three times. You should not feel pain on post-exercise stretching. Always return slowly to the starting position when releasing the stretch.

Below are some examples of stretches that you can do; some whilst sitting, and for those who are happy to stand, there is the standing alternative. Make sure you are in a safe position, i.e. not standing balancing on one leg trying to stretch and balance at the same time. These are a guide only, and if you want to try different ones, there is a wealth of examples on the internet. If you are in any doubt about stretches because of any existing medical condition that you may have, check with your GP or physiotherapist first.

Hamstrings stretch sitting

Put right leg straight out in front of you. Keeping your knee straight, gently slide your right hand down your leg until you feel tension in your hamstrings on the back of your leg. Hold for 30 seconds and then relax. Repeat three times for each leg.

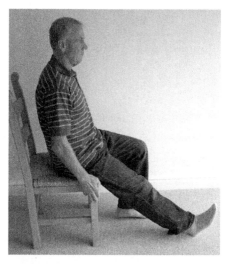

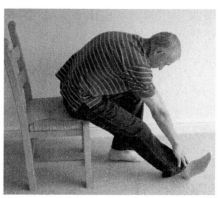

Quads stretch sitting

Sit near the edge of the seat so that your leg can move back along the side of the chair. Hold onto your ankle and gently pull your ankle up and back until you feel the tension in your quads on the front of your thigh. Hold for 30 seconds then relax. Repeat three times for each leg.

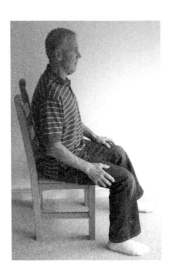 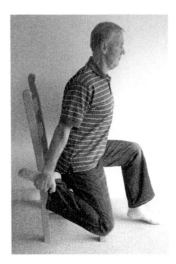

Rotational stretch of your body while sitting

Sit with your back straight and arms folded in front of you. Take your arms round to your left until you feel the tension in your side, back and triceps (back of your arms). Hold for 30 seconds then relax. Repeat three times to each side.

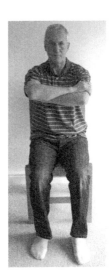 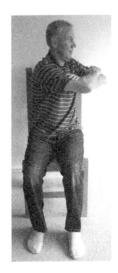 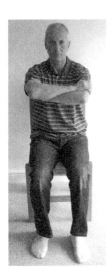

Shoulder stretches while sitting

Reach up as high as you can with both arms until you feel the pull in your arms, shoulders and possibly the sides of your body. Hold for 30 seconds and then relax. Repeat three times.

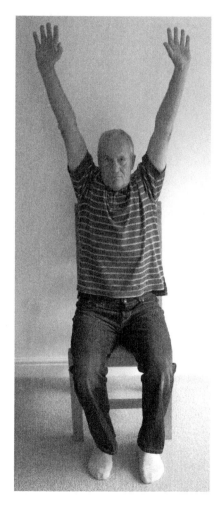

STRETCHES WHILE STANDING

Hamstrings stretch while standing

With your knees straight, slowly lean forwards until you feel tension in your hamstrings on the back of your thighs. Hold for 30 seconds and then relax. Repeat three times. Do not bounce when stretching, and if you feel dizzy do not continue this stretch.

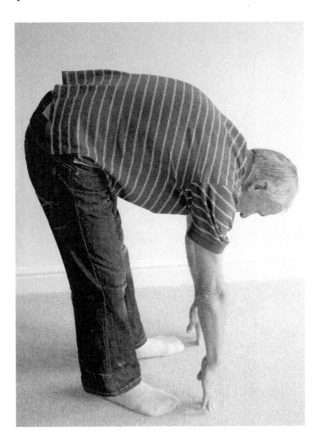

Quads stretch while standing

Whilst holding onto a support for balance with your left hand, pull your right ankle up behind your right hip until you feel the tension in your quads on the front of your thigh. Hold for 30 seconds then relax. Repeat three times for each leg.

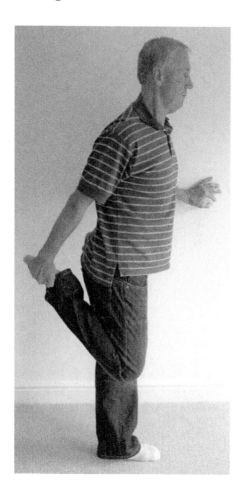

Gastrocs/calf stretch while standing

Stand with your arms straight against a wall and put your left foot forwards knee bent. Keep your right leg back with your heel on the ground and knee straight. Lean forwards against the wall until you feel the tension in your right calf muscle (gastrocs muscle). Hold for 30 seconds and then relax. Repeat three times for each leg.

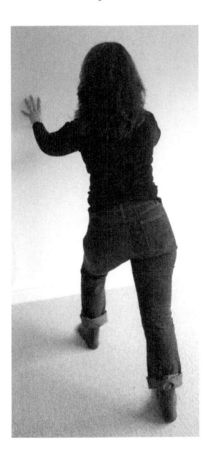

Soleus calf stretch whilst standing

Stand with your arms straight against a wall and put your left foot forwards and knee bent. Place your right leg back but this time with your right knee bent. Lean forwards against the wall until you feel tension in the lower half of your right calf (soleus muscle). Hold for 30 seconds and then relax. Repeat three times for each leg.

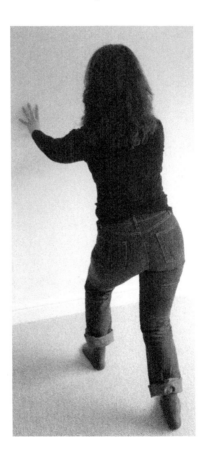

That's it... these are the exercises that work on the specific muscle groups you need and will help you improve your muscle power, be fitter for your golf and so give you the best chance to improve. The exercises and stretches will also help to keep those muscles younger and protect you against injury and arthritis. You just have to get used to fitting them in to your life at least three times a week if possible. With some you will get into the habit of doing them every day which is great. Some you will have to remind yourself to do, but they don't take long and the benefits will be with you for the rest of your life.

WARM UP

Warming up before you play golf is really important to prevent injuries and to generally put less strain on your body. Your golf swing will not work at its best until all of the muscles involved have reached their full flexibility which involves increasing the blood flow to your muscles and joints. This doesn't mean just hitting a few balls up and down the practise driving range and green before starting the round. I mean moving about/ exercising to warm up.

A proper warm-up will get your heart gradually beating faster and increase the temperature of the muscles, allowing them to be more efficient and flexible as you take your joints through their range of movement.

Warming up will also stimulate your nervous system by preparing it to speed up reactions and perform efficient movement, thus producing a better swing.

Most golf players do not want to warm up in front of others. That's fine but not really an excuse not to warm up. Remember, a good warm-up can last up to 40 minutes and can be done at home.

What sort of things should you be doing? I give some ideas here but it is up to you to decide what suits you best. My recommendations are the minimum you should be doing. Again, if in doubt regarding any existing medical condition that you have, check with your GP first.

In order to get your heart rate up and circulating the blood around your body (important for all of the walking you are about to do on the course), you will need to move a bit faster. You could try the following:

- Do high steps (marching) on the spot, gradually increasing your speed

- Run on the spot (gently)

- Go up and down your stairs a few times or just do step-ups on the bottom step

- Once warmed, try 'lunge walking'. To lunge walk, step as far forward as you comfortably can with one leg, hip and knee bent, whilst lifting the heel of your back foot up so that you are on the ball of your back foot. You can just do a single lunge as a stretch, or lunge walking where you are not stretching so far but moving forward as you do it. This gives a little stretch to your legs while your muscles are warm.

- Walk on tip-toe and then on your heels to prepare your calf muscles, tendons and ligaments

- Swing your arms to the sides and above your head

- Rotate your body from one side to the other by looking over your shoulders

- Lastly, do some practise swings, first without your club and then with your club.

This may only take 10 minutes or so but is well worth it to help prevent injuries. Don't ever try to stretch muscles before they have warmed up... it could lead to injury if you do.

COOL DOWN

This is the time to allow your muscles to get rid of any waste products that have developed in them, e.g. lactic acid which can cause soreness after exercise if you don't cool down properly. It is also the time to gently stretch your muscles as they are warm and relaxed following exercise or as soon as you finish on the golf course. Stretches help to realign any small tears of the muscle fibres or ligaments that may have occurred during play. It also helps to maintain the length and flexibility of your muscles, ligaments and all of the soft tissues around your joints. You should stretch before your body cools down, so do it as soon as possible, and ideally less than 10 minutes, after you have played. The longer you leave it the cooler your body gets, and you can injure your muscles if you stretch them when they have cooled down. Do not rush from one stretch to another.

And remember to rehydrate as well after you have played. Think of that as the relaxing part of cooling down. I guess that's what the 19th hole is all about!

CHAPTER 6

HOW TO TREAT AND OVERCOME COMMON GOLF INJURIES, ACHES AND PAINS

The information in this chapter is to help if you are experiencing pain in the areas listed below. It will enable you to understand what to do, and will advise on how long it usually takes for improvement/recovery and any equipment changes that will help.

With the best treatment and the best will in the world, it is not always possible to get rid of pain. Tiger Woods is a prime example. He is very fit, has a team of doctors and physiotherapists working with him, but still suffers with back and knee pain.

Many players continue to play despite their pain or stiffness. This is understandable, and though not always desirable, it is hard to give up the game you love. However, you should not carry on playing if the pain is due to an acute injury. If the pain/stiffness is due to an ongoing medical condition, it may be possible to ease the pain, or accommodate the stiffness, with some simple changes in equipment or technique. I have therefore included, where appropriate, 'what to ask the Pro'. This should help you get the most out of your Pro. The more he/she understands what is causing your limitation, the more he/she will be able to help you adapt your swing to achieve the best outcome possible.

I include information about 'supports and bracing' followed by 'strapping'. Both can be very beneficial for the injured or pain-limited player.

N.B. PRICE (Protection, Rest, Ice, Compression and Elevation treatment) and grade of injury are explained in detail in Chapter 7, in 'How to treat sprains and strains back to match fitness'.

Before applying heat or ice, if you have any circulatory issues, and whether you can take anti-inflammatory drugs, check with your GP.

FOOT

Metatarsalgia: Pain in ball of foot

A fairly common condition, particularly in the ball of the right foot (left foot for left-handed players).

Should you seek medical help? Yes for diagnosis, and if not improved by self-treatment by around 6 weeks you may need an injection.

What self-treatment to use and what is the average recovery time? Follow PRICE treatment, put orthotic insoles with shock absorbing pad in your golf shoes and wear flat shoes with enough width. Hopefully there will be improvement within 2-6 weeks.

What exercises/stretching should you do? Achilles tendon/calf stretch (see stretches in Chapter 5). Exercise your ankle up/down and in circles to maintain mobility.

Are there any changes in swing or equipment that will help? Yes, you could reassess the studs on your golf shoes as you may need to remove or reposition them to relieve pressure through the ball of foot. You may also benefit from putting a pressure absorbing pad in your golf shoe to help overcome the enormous pressure put through this joint during follow-through.

What to ask the Pro:

Pain in the ball of the foot can be caused by the large amount of pressure put through it during follow through. This can result in limiting your follow through.

Many golfers compensate by arching their back to limit the weight going through their right foot (left foot for left-handed players).

To deal with these problems you can ask the Pro, specialist shop or healthcare professional to look at your studs to see if they need adapting or changing to take the pressure off the ball of your foot. You can also ask the Pro to help you change your follow through into a slightly different arc of movement to take the pressure off your foot.

Plantar fasciitis: Pain in heel and/or sole of foot

This condition is often referred to as heel pain and it can gradually get worse over time. Sufferers often experience most pain in the morning or when taking the first step after a period of inactivity. When the band of tissue that runs under the sole of the foot from the heel bone becomes inflamed it is called plantar fasciitis.

Should you seek medical help? Yes for diagnosis, and if not improved by self-treatment after about 6-8 weeks, a referral to a foot specialist may be needed.

What self-treatment to use and what is the average recovery time? You can try putting ice packs (described under Ice treatment in Chapter 7) to the painful area and take pain relief/anti-inflammatories if you are medically allowed to. Some sufferers find wearing a night splint helpful as it prevents tightening of the band of tissue under the foot overnight. It can take up to a year for full recovery, and unfortunately a few people have an ongoing niggling pain for longer, especially if they have not received any treatment for the condition.

What exercises/stretching should you do? Stretching of calf as shown in Chapter 5 but only once the pain has settled. Also see CSP leaflet and NHS choices website for heel pain.*

Are there any changes in swing or equipment that will help? Correctly fitting shoes with an orthotic insole with heel support will help. Some people find that a night splint that is designed to maintain a stretch on your foot through the night can be beneficial, helping to prevent the intense pain felt in the morning.

*see CSP leaflets on foot pain at www.csp.org.uk/publications/exercise-advice-leaflets

Over pronation of foot: rolling inwards of foot

This is when your foot rotates inwards causing fallen arches, foot and knee pain.

Should you seek medical help? Not usually required.

What self-treatment to use and what is the average recovery time? Put good orthotic insoles into your shoes which will instantly improve/correct the problem.

What exercises/stretching should you do? You should exercise the small muscles of the foot by trying to pick up a piece of tissue with your toes. Also stretch your calf muscles (see Chapter 5).

Are there any changes in swing or equipment that will help? Wear supportive shoes with supportive insoles.

Ankle ligaments, Achilles tendon and calf muscle pain

GP/seek medical help: Only for diagnosis if acute injury and severe grade 2 or grade 3 sprain suspected (see Chapter 7) or if pain relief/anti-inflammatory advice needed.

Self-treat and recovery time: For grade 1 and mild grade 2 follow PRICE treatment. Pain relief/anti-inflammatories, as needed. Should be back to full fitness in 4-6 weeks.

Exercise/stretching: Yes, gentle stretching and graded exercises as in table in Chapter 7.

Change in swing or equipment: On impact and follow-through keep left foot slightly outwardly rotated to prevent side pressure on ligaments.

Knee pain: possibly due to arthritis, ligament injury or torn cartilage

GP/seek medical help: Yes for diagnosis, and may need referral to specialist.

Self-treat and recovery time:

- **Arthritis**: ice or heat pack, pain relief as advised by GP, knee support if found beneficial to reduce swelling. Recovery time should see improvement in 6-8 weeks through increased muscle strength.

- **Ligament injury:** PRICE, Pain relief/anti-inflammatories. Should be back to full fitness 4-6 weeks (if grade 1/mild grade 2).

- **Torn cartilage:** PRICE, pain relief/anti-inflammatories. Improvement after 6 weeks if muscles increased in strength but may need surgery to repair damage.

Exercise/stretching:

- **Arthritis:** exercise hip muscles, quads and hamstrings, to support the knee. Stretch to maintain range of movement of joint within pain-free limit as in Chapter 5.

- **Ligament:** yes, as in table for sprains in Chapter 7.

- **Torn cartilage**: as in arthritis above, but will not repair without surgery.

Change in swing or equipment: Use golf ball picker to avoid squatting. Knee support.

What to ask the Pro:

During the impact phase of your swing, up to 80% of your body weight is put through your knees which can initiate pain from an existing condition.

This can affect your swing by making it harder to maintain a stable knee position resulting in a lack of fluid movement through the swing. To help with this, you can ask the Pro to assess you to help achieve a wider stance with your lead foot turned outwards a bit. Also, ask to try a longer shaft as this will reduce the bending and pressure through your knees.

Hip Pain: usually arthritis

GP/seek medical help: Yes, for diagnosis and drug treatment advice.

Self-treat and recovery time: Pain relief/anti-inflammatories. Weight control. Should be some improvement in pain after 6-8 weeks with increased muscle strength.

Exercise/stretching: Yes, to build muscles to support the hip joint and stretches to maintain range of movement of joint as in Chapter 5.

Change in swing or equipment: The classic golf swing (when there is almost equal amounts of shoulder and hip turn) reduces the rotational forces through the hips and spine and so will help decrease pain.

What to ask the Pro:

If you have existing arthritic changes or soft tissue tightness around your hip joint, you may have limited internal rotation (turning inwards) of your hips. This will decrease the speed of your swing. To help alleviate the pain, you can ask the Pro to try a flatter swing with you where the swing plane is more horizontal than the norm. This will decrease the rotational forces through your hips and help decrease the stress through the joint thus decreasing pain.

Back pain

GP/seek medical help: Yes, for diagnosis (as too complicated to self-diagnose) and drug treatment advice. May need referral to specialist.

Self-treat and recovery time: Ice or heat packs, pain relief/anti-inflammatories, posture correction. Recovery time is variable depending on diagnosis, can be 2 weeks to long term.

Exercise/stretching: Yes, gentle exercises and stretching as in Chapter 5 if agreed by GP or appropriate health care professional after diagnosis. Hamstring stretches to relieve tight hamstrings, as they often put stress on lumbar spine. Refer CSP leaflets.

Change in swing or equipment: Slower swing and lighter clubs with softer flex will reduce stress through the back. A more classic swing with less rotation will decrease stress. Longer clubs to prevent bending the spine. You can use a ball-reacher and motorised golf bag. Push the golf trolley, rather than pull it. Supportive lycra garment or soft neoprene wrap may help.

What to ask the Pro:

When playing golf, back pain can be caused by muscle imbalance, weak core muscles, tilting of the pelvis and existing arthritic changes in the spine. Having back pain can result in arching the lower back (hyperextension) during follow-through. Limited rotation of the mid back (thoracic spine) around the pivot point of the swing will result in a shorter swing arc. Neck pain (cervical spine) can result in the incorrect positioning of your head during downswing.

To help with these issues you can ask the Pro to show you how to hit a flatter or classic swing which requires less rotation of the spine so less stress is put through your lower back. Your head position can be assessed to ensure best position to limit stress through your neck. You can ask to try a longer shaft, or a shaft with more flex which will absorb more of the forces transmitted to your body through the shaft.

Shoulder pain

GP/seek medical help: Yes, for diagnosis and drug treatment advice. May need referral to specialist.

Self-treat and recovery time: Yes if minor pain/injury.

- **Arthritis:** pain relief/anti-inflammatories, avoid painful movements and lifting heavy objects.

- **Injury:** as in arthritis, but may also want to refer to CSP leaflets on shoulder injury. Should notice improvement after 6-8 weeks if muscles strengthened.

Exercise/stretching:

- **Arthritis:** gradually increase the amount you are using your arm, gentle pendular exercises to begin with (see CSP leaflets) and build up as described in treatment table, Chapter 7.

- **Injury:** depends on degree of injury, pendular exercises and increased usage as above, but also see diagnosis and treatment tables in Chapter 7. Should be back to full fitness after 4-6 weeks if minor.

Change in swing or equipment: Shorter backswing puts less strain on shoulders. Bend left arm at end of backswing to reduce stress through left shoulder. Gentle follow-through, not excessive, to prevent stress through joint.

What to ask the Pro:

When arthritis, rotator cuff issues or tight soft tissue (stiffness) pain reduces the movement of your shoulder, your backswing becomes limited. Forcing the club through a longer swing can put excessive strain on your shoulder joint. Follow-through can also be limited and forcing it will put strain through your left shoulder (opposite for left-handed players). To prevent this you will need to ask the Pro how to get power in the downswing with limited backswing and how to limit your follow-through. You may also want to talk to your Pro about using lighter clubs as this will lessen the forces going through your shoulders.

Golfer's elbow and wrist pain

GP/seek medical help: Only if unsure of diagnosis or need pain/drug treatment advice or if no improvement in pain after 2 weeks of self-treatment.

Self-treat and recovery time: Yes, ice or heat packs and drug treatment. Pain should ease after 2 weeks, may take 4-6 weeks for full recovery.

Exercise/stretching: Rest initially, avoiding repetitive movements of the arm and hand. Follow guidelines in Chapter 7.

Change in swing or equipment: Reassess grip, may be too small/large. Check wear and tear on gloves as they will show if you are gripping too tightly. Don't use your wrist excessively during your swing. Could use elbow support/splint to redirect forces through your elbow away from inflamed tendon.

What to ask the Pro for elbow pain:

If you are getting pain throughout the swing, but particularly on impact, you may develop a hesitant swing (unsure and indecisive) which can lead to increased muscle tension in your arms and hands. Ask the Pro to check your grip size, that you are not using your wrist excessively, and to try a less stiff shaft which helps to prevent vibrations transmitting to your elbow. Also try not to hit the ball too hard.

What to ask the Pro for wrist pain:

If you are unable to cock your wrist effectively due to pain, you will not be able to generate so much power. Ask the Pro to check your technique, use of your wrist and grip size through the swing.

Supports and bracing

Golf and tennis elbow supports help to ease the stresses travelling through your arm when hitting the ball as they redirect the force through a different part of the tendon, thus reducing the loading of any one part of the tendon. Some players wear the support as a preventative measure and feel more comfortable wearing one than not. That's fine, but with a bit of exercise a support may prevent injury more effectively and/or prevent a different part of the tendon becoming inflamed. Exercises for this are included in Chapter 5, 'Home Exercise Programme'.

I have been asked about knee supports for those experiencing pain in their knees. Firstly, it is important to get a proper diagnosis of what is causing the pain. If a support is required, then it is best to seek professional advice. There are some good knee braces specifically designed for sports players that will off-load some of the pressure through the knee. Neoprene knee supports help to keep the knee warm and some players like that feeling of support, though these won't prevent stress through your joint. They are comfortable to wear and should help prevent swelling of the knee.

Back supports are very difficult to fit so that they do not slip or limit movement when playing golf. You may find that a thin neoprene wrap for the lower back, high lycra shorts or supportive under garments may offer some support and will help keep your soft tissues warm in that area, but these will not prevent over-use or stretching of the soft tissues.

At the end of the day there is no substitute for strong muscles supporting your joints as Mother Nature intended. However, if exercising and strengthening the appropriate muscles isn't enough, bracing may be worth looking into. It is not a short cut, but if it is the best option then you will need professional advice.

Strapping

Many people ask about the latest type of strapping. You will have seen a lot of athletes wearing multi-coloured tape around different parts of the body. There are now many different types of this tape, and the first was called Kinesio tape. It began life in Japan and has taken the world of sport by storm. It is different from the old style of taping that basically protected joints or muscles by limiting their movement as it did not stretch. Kinesio tape is stretchy, and simply put, it allows movement of the muscle and joints. It is thought to 'lift' the skin from the layers beneath allowing better blood flow and *lymphatic drainage*. This means that there is less pressure on the pain nerve ending in the injury sites so pain is decreased. With less pain the body is able to move more normally and so aid the healing process overall. Stiffness because of pain can in itself cause pain, and so it can become a vicious circle and hinder recovery.

Lymphatic drainage: lymph is a fluid that circulates round your body. It has its own system of tubes to flow through that run close to your circulatory system (blood system). It prevents fluid building up in your tissues. When injured we need an efficient lymphatic drainage system to carry the fluid and debris of the injury away. Build-up of fluid in the tissues causes pain.

It is also thought that the tape affects the *fascia* that lies between the different layers of muscles and other soft tissues in your body allowing better drainage, alignment of joints and muscles and so better function and movement.

Fascia: this is a type of connective tissue that surrounds groups and single muscles, blood vessels and nerves. It allows smooth movement between different layers.

The Kinesio tape manufacturers also say that it decreases scar tissue formation and adhesions that can result from injury.

It hasn't taken the place of the old style of taping as that still has a place if immobilisation is required, but it does take the rehab/treatment one step further. At the appropriate stage in the rehabilitation process, it allows the player to go back to their sport with support and free movement, along with the physiological benefits of the taping. The muscle and joints can start to move through the range needed for the sport, limiting any stiffness or occurrence of shortening of soft tissues.

My experience using the tape, and the experience of some of my physiotherapy colleagues, has been very positive and we do use the tape as an additional form of treatment.

Some pharmacies sell pre-cut strapping for the most common injuries which you can apply yourself. This can be of help for minor injuries, but for more serious injuries I would always recommend assessment by a professional before embarking on taping yourself, especially if you have any skin conditions including fragile skin.

CHAPTER 7

HOW TO LOOK AFTER YOURSELF FOLLOWING INJURY

There is a lot you can do for yourself if you get injured. Obviously, this depends on the severity of the injury. You will need to decide if you can treat yourself and be motivated enough to follow the treatment plan and rehabilitation regime to get back to full fitness, or whether you need to be guided through the process by a professional. It is important not to skip corners hoping it will get better on its own. It may take some commitment to get you back to full fitness and prevent further re-injury.

Some people would rather see a physiotherapist if possible, and that would be the best way to get treatment and rehabilitation. You may be able to access a physiotherapist via your GP, or you can go privately. I would advise that if you see a physiotherapist privately, you see one that is registered with the HCPC (Health and Care Professions Council, see website in Chapter 9) which means they are properly qualified and registered.

NHS physiotherapy may not be readily accessible to all for minor injuries and so I will give some basic guidelines. These will inform you as to what the different degrees of injury are, what first aid should be done, and what injury treatment and rehabilitation is needed in order to get back to playing golf.

This is a practical and informative general guide. It cannot replace the expertise/advice that a qualified professional can give you as it is not possible to tailor programmes of treatment to the individual's need in a book. It cannot provide an individual assessment, or take into account any existing medical conditions you may have. The guide therefore has to make the fundamental assumption that there are no existing medical conditions and that the treatment you undertake can only be for minor injuries. If you are at all unsure regarding the extent of the injury or treatment regimes, then I would recommend seeing your GP for a diagnosis and advice regarding which treatment and rehabilitation programmes you should follow.

I will also explain when you should see your GP for any other issues relating to the injury. This is because I have found that some people are reluctant to 'bother' their GP with what they see as a minor ailment. However, your GP is there to help you stay healthy, and it is better for you, and the NHS, if you are able to get back to full fitness and playing your sport as soon as possible. GPs are there to advise you and they know your medical health and what is best for you personally. With this in mind, the guide is not designed to replace any relationship you already have with your GP, hospital specialist or other healthcare professional. It is intended to enable you to understand what usually happens when injury occurs and what to expect through the treatment process. So don't be reluctant to ask if you are in any doubt.

Having said that, I hope this guide will help you, alongside information that you can gain from the NHS Choices website (see below), to do some of the right things and avoid the wrong. The NHS website is a good source of up-to-date information to help keep abreast of any changes in treatment protocols that may happen with further medical research. Having an informed idea regarding the progression of treatment and rehabilitation should help you understand how your injury is recovering, assess your progress and indicate whether you need to seek further advice. It is much better than doing nothing at all. Letting Mother Nature take its course will not repair your injury fully and predisposes you to re-injury. Don't, therefore, try to overlook injuries, as they are part and parcel of the sports player's life, even the minor ones. Let's try to make them a small short-term issue rather than a long-term one.

So what can you do? To start with you need to know about 'first aid'. (Basic information on symptoms, diagnosis, treatment and prevention can also be found on the NHS Choices website www.nhs.uk/conditions/sports-injuries/Pages/Introduction.aspx.)

First aid for minor injuries

Firstly, you need to assess the extent or degree of the injury. Having some idea of what the injury is and the degree of the injury will help you decide whether you need to go straight for medical help or not. If your pain has not improved after following the PRICE treatment below, then you should see your GP.

To enable you to decide the degree of injury, i.e. if it is a mild to moderate, grade 1 or 2 sprain (pulled ligament), or, grade 1 or 2 strain (pulled muscle or tendon), you need to consult the chart below.

If you decide you have a grade 1 or a mild grade 2, you can usually self-treat. If it is a grade 3 sprain or strain (complete rupture) then you need to seek medical help. There is a grey area if you think you have a serious grade 2, and if you are at all unsure of making a judgment on the extent of the injury, you should check with your GP, or other doctor, before going ahead with self-treatment. If you have an Achilles tendon injury, you may want to confirm the grade of injury with a doctor, as sometimes it is difficult for the untrained to diagnose the extent of this particular injury.

You may also experience a lot of pain on initial injury and so may not be able to distinguish a grade 1 injury from a grade 2 at first. However, over the following 36-hour period this should become more apparent as your pain level changes. Even initially, it should be much easier to tell the difference between a grade 1 and grade 3 and this is important as you will need to seek medical advice if you have suffered a grade 3 injury.

Guide to help understand the degree of injury

	Grade 1	Grade 2	Grade 3
Muscle and tendons (Strain) Tendons join muscle to bone	A few fibres stretched or torn. Some pain and tenderness, but should still be able to use it normally	Greater number of fibres torn. More severe pain and tenderness and may be mild swelling and bruising. Some impairment of movement or difficulty weight bearing due to pain	Complete rupture of muscle or tendon. Severe pain and unable to use the muscle, movement severely impaired
Recovery time	Without complications should be pretty well healed in three weeks, full recovery back to sport a bit longer	As in grade 1 with full recovery 4-6 weeks	Can take several months for full rehabilitation
Self-treat or professional	Self-treat	Self-treat, but may want diagnosis confirmed by GP/Doctor	Need professional treatment

	Grade 1	Grade 2	Grade 3
Ligaments (Sprain) Ligaments join bone to bone so are found across joints	Mild stretching of ligament, some pain, tenderness and swelling. May have some difficulty weight bearing	Partial rupture of the ligament, moderate pain. Tenderness and swelling with possible instability of the joint making weight bearing difficult	Complete rupture. Significant pain and swelling, severe impairment of movement. Instability of joint and unable to weight bear
Recovery time	Without complications, should be pretty well healed in three weeks, back to full fitness a little longer	As in grade 1 with full recovery 4-6 weeks	Can take several months for full rehabilitation
Self-treat or professional	Self-treat	Self-treat but may want diagnosis confirmed by GP	Need professional treatment

Don't forget, if in any doubt you should seek professional advice from either your GP or physiotherapist.

Secondly, you need to carry out first aid to the injury. What you do initially after injury can really help speed up recovery and prevent secondary problems. You can't speed up the time it takes your body to heal, but you can give it the best conditions and support to enable the healing process to occur in the most efficient way.

I have mentioned above the first aid regime R.I.C.E or P.R.I.C.E. which stand for:

P = protection

R = rest

I = ice

C = compression

E = elevation

PRICE is the most common treatment regime used by physiotherapists as an initial treatment protocol.

What do all of these treatments do and why should you follow this regime? Let's start with:

Protect/Rest

You need to protect from further injury. As a minimum, you should avoid movements that are in the same direction, or plane, of the injury initially during the acute phase. The **acute phase** can last between 36 and 72 hours and is the immediate post-injury healing phase. It results in inflammation causing pain and swelling. This may mean using some form of support such as crutches if it is a leg injury. Progressive loading of the injury, i.e. gently increasing the movement and pressure through the injury, should begin **after the acute phase and as the pain allows.**

That is to say, try to minimise the amount you move the area of injury for the first 36-72 hours depending on the severity.

> *If after 48 hours of PRICE therapy you are not able to move the injured area or your symptoms are worse, then you should see your GP. If you have noticed any lumps or bumps, or you are still unable to weight bear or if you have pain or tenderness in a different area to where you injured yourself, you should get it checked out by your GP. You should also go if you have any numbness in the injured area. If you are in doubt then get it checked out.*

Ice

You should apply ice to the injured area after a soft tissue injury. The ice provides analgesia (pain relief) to the injured area. It is generally thought that it helps to reduce the swelling and inflammation process that happens following injury. However, this depends on the depth of the injury as our layers of fatty tissue insulate us from the cold and so, depending on the depth, it may not be as effective for these purposes. If the injury is close to the surface of the skin, there may be some effect on swelling, but for deeper structures it is unlikely. It is still recommended in the acute phase, with short regular periods of ice application of around 10-20 minutes, depending on how well it is tolerated, in the first 24-48 hours for pain reduction following injury.

If you have any circulatory or heart conditions then you should check with your GP if you can safely treat yourself with ice.

Do not put ice directly on the skin. You can wrap crushed ice in a damp tea towel and then apply to the injured area. It is also possible to use frozen peas in their bag. The bag of peas should be placed into a second plastic bag (to prevent the pea bag sticking to the skin), then placed on the injury and then covered in a damp towel to keep the cold in. This type of ice treatment is handy and effective, but crushed ice is thought to be more effective.

Compression

Supporting the injured site helps to decrease bleeding and/or swelling and also gives confidence and the feeling of support. Generally, using the appropriate size of doubled-over Tubigrip (or other similar specialist elasticated, tubular, support bandage) will provide an acceptable level of pressure without causing damage. Too much pressure may adversely affect the healing process. It is important to make sure that the Tubigrip/support is not too tight, thus causing numbness or pins and needles. Always follow the manufacturer's guidelines and precautions regarding its sizing, placement and application. Tubigrip is probably the most commonly used elasticated support bandage but others are available. Your local pharmacist will be able to advise you of the options.

Elevation

It is usual to elevate after a soft tissue injury but you should always return the elevated limb to normal position, i.e. gravity dependent position, gradually. It is also best that you do not have a compression garment on while your limb is elevated as this could provide too much pressure on the cells around the injury (interstitial pressure) and hinder the healing process. So take off the compression garment when elevating the limb and put it back on before you return it to a gravity dependent position.

A note on pain relief following injury

It is generally advised that one should take adequate pain relief initially following injury. After 48 hours it may be advisable to take anti-inflammatory drugs, but only if you are medically able to do so.

If you are in any doubt as to what painkillers you are able to take or if you are able to take anti-inflammatory drugs, then you should consult with your GP who will also be able to inform you of the appropriate level of pain relief for your injury. You could also ask your local pharmacist who will be able to advise you on the use of anti-inflammatories and anti-inflammatory gels that you rub into your skin. Many people find these beneficial as they avoid the need for oral drugs.

The next stage after first aid is treatment and rehabilitation. If you go to see a physiotherapist, they will assess the injury, make a diagnosis and then start you on a treatment regime to help control the swelling and limit the pain. Over time they will start to move the joint or muscle and then at the appropriate time of recovery either put weight through your leg if it is a lower limb injury, or use resisted exercise with the arm if it is an upper limb injury. The muscle fibres and collagen fibres of the tendons and ligaments stretch or break when injured. These need to be realigned and strengthened, injured cells to be taken away, new cells formed and the *neural pathways* restored for optimal balance and coordination. This is a really important part of the rehabilitation of sports injuries. These are all things that you can do to help yourself to get back to full fitness for minor injuries.

Neural pathways: *these are the connections from the muscles, tendons and ligaments to the central nervous system and brain which allow the brain to coordinate movement.*

Treatment and rehabilitation

After your first 36-72 hours post injury the first aid stage is over and the treatment stage can begin, assuming there are no complications or factors that may influence recovery.

The more serious the injury, the longer it will take to recover. This may seem obvious, but in my experience, very keen sports players underestimate their injury as they are so eager to get back to their sport. Don't go back until you are fully fit. If you go back too soon, you risk re-injury and a longer rehabilitation time.

I have put together a table as a guide to show you how your treatment should progress. Ideally, you should aim to treat yourself at least three times a day. A little often is usually better than over-doing it, so depending on how you cope with the treatment, see what fits best for you. Remember, this is a practical and informative guide and is not intended as a substitute for professional advice if that is what is needed. It is general guidance and doesn't take into account any particular individual physical or medical condition.

So the treatment/rehabilitation stage for you would mean:

- Start to mobilise (move) the joint or injured muscle (to help realign the torn fibres), and then

- gradually put some weight through the injury, followed at the appropriate stage of recovery by

- starting some exercises to build the muscle through stimulating the production of new muscle fibres.

The following charts will help to guide you through the rehabilitation process of what to do when.

A GUIDE TO TREATMENT PROGRESSION OF MINOR 'SPRAINS AND STRAINS' OF THE LEG

Initial treatment in the first 36-72 hours

	First 36-72 hours
Walking/taking weight through your leg	Rest, you may need crutches
Exercise	Not until at least 48 hours after injury and then depends on level of pain
Balance work	Not yet
Stretching (on warmed muscles)	Not yet
Ice and/or pain relief	**Yes***

*you must check with your GP that you are safe to put ice on your leg if you have any diabetic or circulatory problems.

Treatment 3-6 days after injury (repair of torn fibres phase)

	3-6 days post injury
Walking/taking weight through your leg	**Yes** (supported with crutches if necessary until pain decreases). Wear compression when standing, e.g. Tubigrip
Exercise	**Yes.** Gently start to move muscle/joint. Gently progress to full *range of movement* as pain allows without standing on it (*weight bearing through it*). When standing ensure Tubigrip is on and only put amount of weight through as pain allows.
Balance exercises	Not yet
Stretching (on warmed muscles)*	Very gently take muscle/joint to end of range of movement, hold for 10 seconds and then relax.
Ice and/or pain relief	**Yes** as required

*you should only stretch a muscle when it has warmed up, i.e. you need to take it through its non-painful range of movement several times before stretching. That means that the blood flow has increased to the muscle and warmed it up.

Between the **6 days and the 4 week** timeframe, as you begin to take weight through your leg again, start to gradually increase your functional activities, i.e. getting out of a chair without holding on, going up and down stairs, step ups (see exercises in Chapter 5). Walking up and down slopes is a simple way to increase the resistance placed on the muscles. You can gradually increase the resistance by walking up/down slopes with greater inclines. Only increase the amount of resistance, repetitions and speed of the exercises slowly, and within pain tolerance, until you have reached your pre-injury level at around 4-6 weeks.

Treatment 4-6 weeks post injury

	By 4-6 weeks depending on extent of injury (more severe ligament and tendon injuries may take longer)
Walking/ taking weight through your leg	**Yes.** You should be fully mobile. There may still be fibres repairing for up to 6 weeks, so depending on the severity, if you are strong enough in the repair, you should be able to start running.
Exercise	**Yes.** You should now be able to take your whole body weight through your leg when standing on one leg. **For calf injury,** you should be able to stand on tip toes and go up and down whilst holding onto a support. **For hamstring injury**, you should be able to stand on injured leg and bend knee then straighten whilst holding onto a support. For both injuries, no support (i.e. crutches) should be required. Gently start exercises in home exercise programme.

Balance work	**Yes.** By 6 weeks you should be able to stand on one leg, balance whilst throwing a ball at the wall and catching it. If you want to progress this then use a balance/wobble board.*
Stretching (on warmed muscles)	**Yes.** You should be able to do a full stretch of the muscle group (of injured muscle or around injured ligament or tendon). Remember always to stretch when your muscles are warmed up. Always stretch after play or exercise to maintain range of movement, flexibility and to prevent scar tissue mal-alignment.
Ice and/or pain relief	Shouldn't need pain relief or ice by now. You should see your GP if still experiencing pain.

*to see what a balance board or wobble board is, look on the website, www.physioroom. com and search 'wobble boards'.

What is range of movement? *This is the natural, or normal amount of movement that a joint or muscle can move through before injury.* **End of range of movement***: This is the end of the natural or normal range of movement that a joint or muscle can be taken through. Moving it past this point will normally cause injury.*

Weight bearing: *This is when you put some weight through the limb. For legs it would be standing on the leg and allowing weight to go through it. For arms it would mean leaning some weight through your arm.*

For specific exercises for knee pain look at the Chartered Society of Physiotherapy website www.csp.org.uk/publications/exercise-advice-leaflets

You can also seek advice on the NHS Choices website.

Tip: If you have suffered an injury to your calf muscles or Achilles tendon, you may find it helpful initially to put a small wedge in your shoe under your heel on that side. This will take some of the stretch and pressure off your calf when standing and walking on it. It effectively decreases the distance the muscles/tendon has to go through to touch the ground.

INJURIES OF THE ARM/SHOULDER

A guide to show treatment progression of minor 'sprains and strains' of the arm and shoulder

	First 36-72 hours post injury
Move or rest	Rest
Exercises	None
Functional activities	None that involve lifting any weight, and only move within limits of pain
Stretching	None
Ice and/or pain relief	**Yes** *

*You must check with your GP before putting ice on if you have any circulatory or heart problems.

	3-6 days (repair of fibres phase)
Move or rest	Start gentle exercises
Exercises	Gently start to move with *pendular exercises** then gradually progress to lifting arm as pain allows
Functional activities	Start to reuse with daily activities as pain allows
Stretching	Very gently move as far as you can but avoid movements that cause pain
Ice and/or pain relief	**Yes**, ice optional

*see below, or refer to the Physiotherapy (CSP) advice leaflets for shoulder exercises, link given on page 158

	6 days onwards
Move or rest	Do exercises
Exercises	Gradually start adding weights to lift as pain allows, e.g. can of beans
Functional activities	Try to use as normally as possible but without lifting heavy weights
Stretching	Continue to take it through its range of movement as above (for 3-6 days)
Ice and/or pain relief	**Yes**, may not need ice now and may require less pain relief

	By 4-6 weeks, depending on extent of injury. More severe ligament and tendon injuries can take longer
Move or rest	No rest needed
Exercises	Working to full range of movement with amount of weights you would lift each day pre injury
Functional activities	Use for all of your regular daily activities and start going through range of movement for your golf swing. Hit some balls to assess how pain is.
Stretching	Take through range of movement after exercise when muscles are warmed. Hold at end of range of movement for 30 seconds.
Ice and/or pain relief	**Yes** as needed but should be less now. If pain is no better and you still require pain relief then see GP or physiotherapist.

Pendular exercises: these exercises use the weight of your arm to allow movement at the shoulder. You need to bend forwards at the waist so that your back is parallel to the floor, holding onto a table or chair for support. Let your arm hang downwards and then swing it forwards, backwards and in circles depending on the movement required.

When you are able to start gentle exercises I would recommend reading the Chartered Society of Physiotherapy guidelines for shoulder pain or tennis elbow (as appropriate to your injury). You can find the guidelines by going to the Chartered Society of Physiotherapy (CSP) website and downloading the relevant guide. The link is:

www.csp.org.uk/publications/exercise-advice-leaflets

I haven't said anything about back injuries in this section as they are very complicated, difficult to diagnose and professional advice should be sought before you try to self-treat. I would recommend that you see the appropriate healthcare professional if you are experiencing back pain. You can look up the advice leaflet given by The Chartered Society of Physiotherapy (CSP) (see above).

Finally, once you have treated your injury and you are well on the road to recovery, you must not forget one of the most important aspects of a rehabilitation programme for a sports player. This is to work on balance, coordination and joint position sense following injury.

This is important because when injured, it is not only the muscle fibres and collagen fibres of the tendons and ligaments that become stretched or break, the receptors in these structures that provide continuous feedback to the brain regarding their state of stretch and joint position are also affected. In other words, the connections from the muscles and ligaments to the brain are affected and need to be restored for full function/fitness to be achieved. This is where the correct rehabilitation is essential, and, unless directed by a professional, is often overlooked when rehabilitating oneself back to playing again.

This feedback is provided by specialist cells throughout our bodies, but to keep it simple, I am only referring to the ones in our ligaments and muscles. These provide the body with the necessary joint position sense, proprioception and kinaesthesia to enable good balance and coordination. Without joint position sense, our brains cannot react quickly enough to prevent us losing balance, and cannot correct us in time to prevent re-injury. So, yes, do your first aid, do the graduated exercises to get back the strength and flexibility, but do not forget the balance and coordination work when at the appropriate stage of recovery.

To summarise the main points of general treatment following minor injury:

- Apply appropriate first aid for the first 36-72 hours depending on severity of the injury (PRICE).

- Start to move and exercise from 3-6 days onwards, as advised, to help realign the muscle fibres and facilitate the repair process.

- Manage your pain, as pain can cause muscle spasm which can be detrimental to healing. However, if you use pain killers to decrease pain, remember that you are injured so don't overdo it.

- Gradually work on balance and coordination when able to weight bear fully through the limb.

- Rehabilitate by working through the movement patterns that are needed to perform your golf swing with the appropriate muscle strengthening and flexibility.

- If you do not think you are making the progress that you should be, see your GP or physiotherapist for advice, as getting it right now will help prevent re-injury.

NB: This is assuming that there are no complications, existing medical conditions and that you have consulted the appropriate healthcare professional, NHS website or other authoritative information sites if you are in any doubt.

CHAPTER 8

PERSONAL EXERCISE RECORD

These tables can also be downloaded from my website
www.fitterforever.org

Lying

Exercise	Week 1 Sets/reps	Week 2 Sets/reps	Week 3 Sets/reps	Week 4 Sets/reps	Week 5 Sets/reps	Week 6 Sets/reps	Week 7 Sets/reps	Week 8 Sets/reps
knee rolling								
back arching / rounding								
hip rotation								

Sitting

Exercise	Week 1 Sets/reps	Week 2 Sets/reps	Week 3 Sets/reps	Week 4 Sets/reps	Week 5 Sets/reps	Week 6 Sets/reps	Week 7 Sets/reps	Week 8 Sets/reps
wrist								
arms apart								
overhead								
band over door								
diagonal pull to left								
to right								
sitting / standing								

Standing

Exercise	Week 1 Sets/reps	Week 2 Sets/reps	Week 3 Sets/reps	Week 4 Sets/reps	Week 5 Sets/reps	Week 6 Sets/reps	Week 7 Sets/reps	Week 8 Sets/reps
right knee dip								
left knee dip								
lift heels up								
sit to stand practise								

Exercise using your stairs

Exercise	Week 1 Sets/reps	Week 2 Sets/reps	Week 3 Sets/reps	Week 4 Sets/reps	Week 5 Sets/reps	Week 6 Sets/reps	Week 7 Sets/reps	Week 8 Sets/reps
2 steps at a time								
step ups right								
step ups left								
with weights								

Balance exercises

Exercise	Week 1 Sets/reps	Week 2 Sets/reps	Week 3 Sets/reps	Week 4 Sets/reps	Week 5 Sets/reps	Week 6 Sets/reps	Week 7 Sets/reps	Week 8 Sets/reps
balance when brushing teeth								
eyes open/ closed								

Advanced exercises

Exercise	Week 1 Sets/reps	Week 2 Sets/reps	Week 3 Sets/reps	Week 4 Sets/reps	Week 5 Sets/reps	Week 6 Sets/reps	Week 7 Sets/reps	Week 8 Sets/reps
advanced arm lift straight								
advanced arm lift with rotation								

CHAPTER 9

EQUIPMENT AND USEFUL WEBSITES

Elastic resistive bands

Theraband is one of the largest companies supplying the elastic resistance exercise bands that I use for my exercise programme. They produce a range of bands with varying degrees of resistance that you can work through when increasing your strength.

The website link is: www.thera-bands.co.uk/index.php

On their website you will see they have a range of products that may interest you. The resistance bands are coloured in order of their resistance, yellow being the easiest, gold the hardest. The colour order is:

Yellow, red, green, blue, black, silver and gold.

I find that women tend to use the red to black and men the blue to gold. It all depends on your strength and how far you are through your exercise building regime. It also depends on which muscle groups you are working as your legs are stronger than your arms, so you may need a higher resistance band for your legs.

Many other companies supply elasticated resistance bands. I have listed a few that are on the internet but there are many others if you search for them. I have seen that my local large supermarket and sports shop sell sets of bands.

When buying bands, check what resistance the colour represents as this may vary from company to company but the same principles apply, lower resistance for weaker muscles.

www.thera-bands.co.uk
www.amazon.co.uk
www.physiosupplies.com
www.ebay.co.uk
www.return2fitness.co.uk
www.physioroom.com
www.boots.co.uk
www.jpmproducts.co.uk

If you go to the Theraband website home page you will be able to download their free booklet that gives all of the information you will need regarding safety and care of your bands and, if you are interested in having a look at other exercise options, a range of exercises for each muscle group with instructions.

I recommend that you read the precautions and care of your band before use.

When buying a length of banding I suggest that you need a minimum of 1.5 metres to get full use out of the band. It will enable you to make a loop out of it or double it over to increase the resistance.

Exercise weights

These can be purchased from sports shops, the larger supermarkets and online. I recommend starting with ankle weights which are usually 2.5 kg, and you can use them in your hands as well as around your legs.

General health advice

Go to the NHS website for information:
www.nhs.uk/Conditions/Pages/hub.aspx

Physiotherapy advice leaflets

The Chartered Society of Physiotherapy has produced a series of information leaflets that you can download from their website to give you information regarding self-treatment and exercises for some of the common pains and injuries. They are well worth looking at. The leaflets are on: foot pain, carpal tunnel syndrome, knee pain, neck pain, shoulder pain, tennis elbow and back pain.

The website link is: www.csp.org.uk/publications/exercise-advice-leaflets

Podiatry for foot issues

The professional body for podiatrists have information regarding all sorts of foot problems. Their website is: www.scpod.org

Dieticians for diet and healthy eating advice

The professional body for dieticians has a lot of information that the public can access on their website which is: www.bda.uk.com

Orthotics for splints and footwear advice

Contact details and information regarding services provided by orthotists is provided on their website: www.bapo.com

The Health and Care Professions Council

You can go to this website to check that the healthcare professional is registered with them. The website is: www.hpc-uk.org

For more information, please visit my website: www.Fitterforever.org for updates, exercise record downloads and a whole lot more!

ABOUT THE AUTHOR

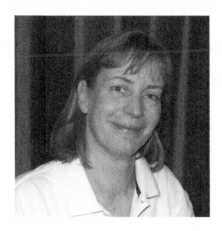

Suzanne Clark established Fitter Forever, an organisation that helps people over 50 stay fit and healthy enough to continue playing sport as they get older. She is an all-round sports player, including adventurous activities such as sprint triathlons, off-piste skiing and sailing around the UK coast.

Suzanne is a member of the Chartered Society of Physiotherapy and is registered with the Health and Care Professions Council.